Clinical Guidelines
and Care Protocols

Clinical Guidelines and Care Protocols

Jaqui Hewitt-Taylor PhD BA(HONS) RSCN RGN
*Practice Development Fellow, Institute of Health and
Community Studies, Bournemouth University, UK*

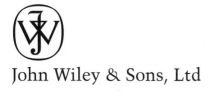

John Wiley & Sons, Ltd

Copyright © 2006   Whurr Publishers Limited (a subsidiary of John Wiley & Sons Ltd)
The Atrium, Southern Gate, Chichester,
West Sussex PO19 8SQ, England
Telephone (+44) 1243 779777

Email (for orders and customer service enquiries): cs-books@wiley.co.uk
Visit our Home Page on www.wiley.com

Other Wiley Editorial Offices

John Wiley & Sons Inc., 111 River Street, Hoboken, NJ 07030, USA

Jossey-Bass, 989 Market Street, San Francisco, CA 94103-1741, USA

Wiley-VCH Verlag GmbH, Boschstr. 12, D-69469 Weinheim, Germany

John Wiley & Sons Australia Ltd, 42 McDougall Street, Milton, Queensland 4064, Australia

John Wiley & Sons (Asia) Pte Ltd, 2 Clementi Loop #02-01, Jin Xing Distripark, Singapore 129809

John Wiley & Sons Canada Ltd, 22 Worcester Road, Etobicoke, Ontario, Canada M9W 1L1

Wiley also publishes its books in a variety of electronic formats. Some content that appears in print may not be available in electronic books.

Library of Congress Cataloging-in-Publication Date
Hewitt-Taylor, Jaqui
    Clinical guidelines and care protocols / Jaquelina Hewitt–Taylor.
        p.   ;   cm.
    Includes bibliographical references.
    ISBN 0-470-01982-4
    1. Medical protocols.   2. Clinical medicine – Standards.   3. Evidence-based medicine.
I. Title.
    [DNLM: 1. Practice Guidelines.   2. Clinical Protocols.   3. Evidence-Based Medicine.
W 84.1 H611c 2006]
RC64.H49 2006
362.1′068 – dc22

2005036435

British Library Cataloguing in Publication Data
A catalogue record for this book is available from the British Library

ISBN-13   978-0-470-01982-5
ISBN-10   0-470-01982-4

Printed and bound in Great Britain by TJ International Ltd, Padstow, Cornwall
This book is printed on acid-free paper responsibly manufactured from sustainable forestry in which at least two trees are planted for each one used for paper production.

For my nine-month-old son, John, who taught me that you can type a manuscript one-handed if you need to, and that reference lists make good eating.

Contents

List of Abbreviations

AGREE – Appraisal of Guidelines, Research and Evaluation
DoH – Department of Health
CRD – Centre for Reviews and Dissemination
GMC – General Medical Council
NCC – National Collaborating Centre
NHS – National Health Service
NICE – National Institute of Clinical Excellence
NMC – Nursing and Midwifery Council
PALS – Patients' Advisory and Liaison Services
QALYs – Quality Adjusted Life Years
RCT – randomised controlled trial
RCN – Royal College of Nursing (out in full p. 135)
SHO – senior house officer
SIGN – Scottish Intercollegiate Guideline Network
SpR – specialist registrar
UKCC – United Kingdom Central Council for Nursing, Midwifery and Health
    Visiting (now the Nursing and Midwifery Council)

1
Evidence-based Practice, Clinical Guidelines and Care Protocols

The increasing focus on the use of clinical guidelines and care protocols in healthcare has coincided with an emphasis on evidence-based practice. Evidence-based practice should mean that practice is guided by the best, most up-to-date information on the optimum way to provide care, rather than being based on tradition, habit or the unsubstantiated preferences of individual practitioners (DoH, 2000). It is linked with clinical guidelines and care protocols in so far as clinical guidelines and care protocols should be developed from the current best evidence regarding the aspects of care that they address. They are therefore a tool which practitioners may be able to use in order to base care on the current best evidence.

In order to understand the issues involved in using clinical guidelines and care protocols it is therefore useful to begin by considering the principles that underpin the concept of evidence-based practice. This chapter will discuss what evidence-based practice is, how the current emphasis on evidence-based practice has developed and some of the professional and political aspects of this.

EVIDENCE-BASED PRACTICE

One of the most commonly used definitions of evidence-based practice is that of Sackett *et al.* (1996). They define evidence-based practice as:

> The conscientious, explicit and judicious use of current best evidence in making decisions about the care of individual patients.

They also state that:

The practice of evidence-based medicine means integrating individual expertise with the best available external clinical evidence from systematic research.

Evidence-based practice has also been defined as:

The process by which nurses make clinical decisions using the best available research evidence, their clinical expertise and patient preferences, in the context of available resources. (Di Censo *et al.*, 1998).

A major influencing factor in the increasing popularity of the term 'evidence-based practice' has been the concern over the use of practices that appear to be based on tradition, habit or the unsubstantiated preferences of individuals rather than evidence of their efficacy. Evidence-based practice has been distinguished from these approaches because, as the definitions above show, it seeks to provide treatment, care or interventions based on the evidence of their effectiveness.

Tradition can be defined as 'the transmission of customs or beliefs from generation to generation' (Oxford English Dictionary, 2001). Practice which has become established by tradition, or which is based on the personal preferences of healthcare staff is not necessarily wrong or unsafe. When the evidence regarding an intervention is collected, evaluated and synthesised, it may be clear that an approach which has been used for many years is the best. Logically, this is likely to be so in many cases, because something which works well is likely to become established practice.

I have used the same travel company to book flights since 1997 because they generally seem to have had the best price for what I want. I usually check three or four companies' prices, but, because I have become used to this company having the best deal, I do not always check as diligently as I might that they definitely have the best fares. This year, in a moment of post-natal economising against the day when my nine-month-old son realises that 'hand me down' is not actually a designer label, I undertook a thorough investigation of prices. My usual company still had the best deal for flight prices. They also had the best price for my 'supplement'. (Travel companies refer to my baby as a 'supplement' so as to justify his 'free' flight to the USA costing at least £70.) My established practice was vindicated after a very thorough search of the evidence and I continued to use this company. However, while established practice may be based on what was once best, and may still produce the best results, this may not always be the case. Another company might have had a better deal for my supplement and me. The distinction between established practice and evidence-based practice is that in evidence-based practice the efficacy of established practice in comparison to other currently available approaches is questioned and whether it is really the best approach, or still the best approach, is determined.

An approach to care provision may have been used with apparent success for many years, but evidence-based practice would demand that the reason for its apparent effectiveness be explored and that other approaches which might be more effective be considered. An intervention may appear to be successful, and may to an extent be successful, but, when it is compared to alternatives, it may be evident that another option might be even more effective. My usual company's best offer for a flight from London to San Francisco was £807 for two adults and one supplement, including all those airport taxes that can add a hundred pounds to your holiday costs when you're not looking. This seemed quite a good price, especially as it was at the end of the school holiday/very expensive season, but before I committed my credit card details I felt the need to check that no one could make me a better offer. In the same way, evidence-based practice may not mean that established practice must be changed, but its worth in relation to the alternatives must be demonstrated before its continued use can be approved.

Evidence-based practice also requires practice to be based on the **current** best evidence. A certain approach to care may once have constituted best practice, but developments since its original inception may mean that better methods now exist. For example, developments in scientific knowledge and technology mean that the best way to provide and manage assisted ventilation in neonates has altered over the years. Changes in the dominant beliefs and values of society may also alter what is perceived to be best practice. It was once seen as being in patients' best interests to have decisions made on their behalf by healthcare professionals. However, this view is now seen as outmoded, and in most cases inappropriate. Best practice now requires patients to be involved in the decision-making processes regarding their health (Kennedy, 2003). Thus, basing practice on what was once the best method of care or the most appropriate intervention may no longer represent high-quality care or best practice.

New evidence may also emerge which indicates that an approach to care which was once considered optimum is in fact not safe and should be discontinued. For example, a drug may be found to have adverse effects which mean that its continued use cannot be recommended. In 2001, the National Institute of Clinical Excellence (NICE) made recommendations on the use of selective Cox-2 inhibitors for the treatment of osteoarthritis and rheumatoid arthritis (NICE, 2001a). In late 2004, Vioxx (rofecoxib), one of the drugs in this group, was withdrawn by the manufacturer as it had been found to be strongly associated with the development of heart disease and stroke. NICE are therefore reviewing their guidance on the use of selective Cox-2 inhibitors and so the previous guidance has been suspended (NICE, 2005a). In this instance, at the time of publication, NICE's guidance on the use of these drugs was based on the best available evidence, but new evidence suggests that following the original guidance would not be appropriate.

For best practice to occur, the evidence used to inform practice must therefore be up to date. Although this seems an irrefutable statement, given the speed with which knowledge advances it is often difficult for staff to keep abreast of all the developments in their field of practice (Bates *et al.*, 2003). Even within a very clearly delineated area of practice, keeping up to date with all the information on every area of practice can be a challenge. The care of even a single patient within a speciality requires a range of knowledge to be drawn on. Caring for a person who has Systemic Lupus Erythematous requires knowledge of physiology and pathophysiology which may span a number of systems and specialities. This includes the musculoskeletal system, renal system, nervous system, respiratory system, cardiovascular system, skin and gastrointestinal system and associated clinical specialities. Knowing about the possible effects of this disease on these systems, the treatment and interventions which are recommended, the likely side effects and complications of these and how they may affect and be affected by one another requires a significant range of knowledge. To provide for all of a patient with Lupus' needs, this must be accompanied by an awareness of a range of other aspects of care, such as psychosocial issues and the management of acute and chronic pain and fatigue. The work involved in remaining up to date in all aspects of the care of this one patient is considerable, but to expand this to remaining up to date in all aspects of care for all patients in a rheumatology department would be an even greater challenge. One advantage of clinical guidelines and care protocols is that they can be useful summaries of the current best evidence. This may be a realistic way to enable professionals to access the current best evidence on a range of aspects of care. It nonetheless relies on the guidelines themselves being derived from high-quality, up-to-date evidence.

Evidence-based practice is therefore practice which is carried out in accordance with the current best evidence. Chapter 2 considers what constitutes evidence and the relative importance attributed to different types of evidence. However, there is more to evidence-based practice than finding and then using research on a subject. The definitions by Sackett *et al.* (1996) and Di Censo *et al.* (1998) indicate that the evidence which is used to inform practice should include a variety of sources: research, clinical expertise, patients' views and cost. Evidence, in the context of evidence-based practice, also includes the evidence from the perspectives of healthcare professionals, patients and health economists. It is clear from this that I am not an evidence-based traveller. I mostly consider cost, have a preference for Singapore Airlines for Australasian flights, a complete bias for Aerolíneas Argentinas for flying to Argentina, but otherwise anything with the right number of wings and enough engines for comfort will do. My airline booking practice is based on evidence of cost, and a bit of personal preference, not evidence of the relative merits of the flight path, the airline company, the efficacy of the type of plane involved or the total quality per pound spent in relation to standard of meals, smileyness of staff and whatever else might contribute to quality in airline travel. In this book, the place which cost occupies in healthcare will be a recurrent theme, and my approach to cost in airline travel is not the recommended approach in healthcare.

MORE THAN RESEARCH

Research is an important part of the evidence that should inform practice, but there is more to evidence-based practice than finding research about an aspect of care and making recommendations for practice from this. First of all, evidence-based practice avoids reliance on a single piece of research. In evidence-based practice, all the research on a subject, not just one piece, should be considered. Secondly, in evidence-based practice, research is seen as one form of evidence, and is therefore considered in conjunction with other types of evidence. In evidence-based practice, all the available evidence is gathered, evaluated and synthesised to determine what the recommendations should be. For evidence-based *practice* to occur, these recommendations must be used appropriately in practice. This last point is arguably the most important: that evidence must move beyond the theoretical to the real world of patient care.

The *Kennedy Report* (Kennedy, 2001) identifies that for evidence about healthcare to be beneficial to patients it must be made clinically applicable and used appropriately. Research findings are often not used to their full potential because they are not explained in terms that make the way in which they can be used in practice clear (Bell, 2003; Stewart, 2003). This is sometimes because the research is not intended to be immediately applied to practice. Research about fluid dynamics may ultimately make a valuable contribution to many clinical situations, such as haemodialysis or the administration of intravenous infusions. However, the implications of such research in its raw state are unlikely to be evident to the average practitioner and are not intended to be immediately translated into clinical practice. This type of information requires further stages of interpretation and application of its findings before they can be applied to healthcare practice. Some forms of medical research which are more directly linked to patient care may also require interpretation and explanation before they can be used by the majority of practitioners. For example, Stewart (2003) suggests that despite the undoubted importance of discoveries related to genetics and other aspects of cellular biology it is often difficult for practitioners to know what the everyday practical implications of this new knowledge are.

One of the intentions of evidence-based practice is that, as its name suggests, it is practice based on evidence, not evidence that is recorded in theses, scientific reports or articles but not used. For evidence-based practice to occur, its importance and application to specific clinical situations need to be apparent to clinical staff. For example, while there exists a body of knowledge based on research about the various types of scanning (MRI, CT and PET) available to clinicians regarding how each technique works, the types of image produced, the accuracy of images for various tissue types and what different imaging techniques show about various organs, evidence-based practice might help the clinician to decide which is preferable in a given situation – for example immediately post head injury – and why.

There is an argument that practitioners should be able to identify for themselves the clinical implications of research that has been conducted in their field of practice. While this would, ideally, be the case, it may be an overly optimistic view. As identified above, not all research is designed for immediate clinical application. Even when it is, healthcare staff may not always be able to see how it applies to their practice. This may be either because the research report does not make this clear or because healthcare staff are not all used to reading such reports. Bergus *et al.* (2004) found that most students completing medical school could appraise an article about a diagnostic test but that few could apply the findings to practice. This supports the suggestion that information alone, and especially academic articles or research reports, may not of itself, be enough to influence practice, even when it can be understood in abstract terms. In other cases, individuals may be able to see the clinical application of reports but be less confident that they are based on good evidence. Healthcare is provided by a range of staff, whose skills and confidence in reading and interpreting research reports, and identifying how this applies to practice, will vary. This is aside from the time that it takes to read and interpret such reports and from the fact that not all reports present good-quality information. The volume of information which is available makes it unlikely that all staff in any speciality will be able read, evaluate and consider the practical implications of all the evidence in their field.

It is likely to be useful for the practical implications of research to be clarified so that it can be used appropriately by all the staff who provide care. This is one reason why clinical guidelines that summarise the current best evidence and provide information on its practical application may be useful.

One of the desirable differences between evidence-based practice and abstract research is that evidence-based practice should be grounded in reality, and thus avoid the gap between theory and practice which has often led to problems with implementing research findings (Berenholtz and Pronovost, 2003). This means that the evidence should include whether the findings from research will be practicable or not and how they can be put into practice, as well as their apparent value. Incorporating expert opinion and patient preferences in the evidence used is likely to be beneficial in this respect. This includes using any documented evidence of the practicality of suggested interventions but also seeking advice as to whether suggestions which are made from an evaluation of the evidence are likely to be workable, and acceptable, to users of the service. This includes those who will use them, such as healthcare staff, and patients who will receive care. Recommendations from research which show what is 'best' may give recommendations that involve impractical procedures for staff or steps such as prolonged or invasive treatment or significant travel to lead centres, which may be unacceptable to patients. Thus, potential users of the research may disregard it, irrespective of the quality of the research and its intrinsic potential to improve healthcare.

An example of where advice from experts, and in particular one Professor Herrero, was deemed impractical in a real-world situation comes from Bill Bryson's (1997) preparations for a hike amongst bears on the Appalachian Trail. He notes: 'All the books tell you that if a grizzly comes for you, on no account should you run. This is the sort of advice that you get from someone who is sitting at a keyboard when he gives it.' Bryson goes on to conclude that: 'if you are in an open space and a grizzly comes for you, run. You may as well. If nothing else, it will give you something to do with the last seven seconds of your life.' Later on, he notes that: 'To ward off an aggressive black bear, (Professor) Herrero suggests making lots of noise, banging pots and pans together, throwing sticks and "running at the bear". (Yeah, right, you first, professor.)' (Bryson, 1997).

Bill, it seems, not only found the advice a tad confusing but believed that it would not be very practical in a real-world situation when confronted with a real-world bear.

The aim of the documents which are produced to support evidence-based practice, such as clinical guidelines, is therefore to present practitioners with the best available evidence and to indicate how this applies to practice, and for this to have been devised in such a way that it will be workable in a real-world situation, not just in theory.

However, for evidence-based practice to occur, the evidence that is presented should not only be used but be used in conjunction with individual clinical expertise and patient choice (Sackett *et al.*, 1996; Di Censo *et al.*, 1998; Drake *et al.*, 2004). Going back to my baby-kit purchasing nightmare, I have finally conceded to the need for a wheeled vehicle to transport John. He now weighs in at about ten kilos. I used to carry him in one of those BABY-BJORN front-carrier things, and now that he is bigger I usually carry him in a backpack. This is fine, but it isn't much good when you need to put your shopping in a backpack too. The backpack has a little bag with it, which can take six or so extra kilos, but the staff in our local stores all get very nervous when I put a few kilos of shopping in, and then casually swing the backpack containing a few veggies and the baby upwards. I think I have seen a plain-clothes police officer from the child protection team standing by. So, because I still need my professional registration, I have been obliged to procure a buggy.

All I want to do is put John in it, wheel him to the stores, buy a few potatoes and then take him home and fold it up small, because there is no space for anything in the house. Occasionally, if I am feeling lazy and can't be bothered biking longer distances, I may wish to hop on a bus or train, and so I want it to be lightweight and easy to fold, because I always decide to get on a bus at the last minute and don't have time for lots of folding. From all the reports on safety, comfort, extra fun things you can do with a buggy except carry a child in it, the £300-plus range of buggies are undoubtedly the best. However, for me, they are not worth the money because I want lightweight, compact and easy folding and John is disinclined to live in a buggy. By a happy coincidence such an item is available for only £17.50 from Toys 'R' Us. No doubt the advice on buying a more expensive buggy is good, and developed with input from experts in the field and users of buggies, but for me, the best option is the no-frills, small, lightweight and easy-folding model. It is also so cheap and nasty looking that if John has any desire for street cred his walking ability will progress rapidly.

Likewise in healthcare, although any guidance developed should incorporate expert opinion and patients' views, it is still incumbent on individual practitioners to determine how far this evidence is applicable in each specific situation. Wherever possible, this should be decided in conjunction with the recipient of care. There may be circumstances in which this is not possible, for example a patient who is critically ill may be unable to respond in any way during the most severe stage of their illness. However, in most cases the patient's preferences regarding treatment should be ascertained. If I had been presented with a top-of-the-range buggy and a bill for £300 by a well-meaning do-gooder, I would not have been impressed, however good the evidence they had acted on. Chapter 2 discusses the ways in which professional expertise and patient preferences can be included in the evidence which informs practice, and Chapters 8 and 9 explore in more detail the concept of professional expertise and patient choices in relation to clinical guidelines and care protocols. Both are a vital part of evidence-based practice.

Evidence-based practice means using evidence in the real world of healthcare. Cost is a reality of healthcare and therefore forms a part of the evidence which should inform real-world practice (Sackett *et al.*, 1996; Di Censo *et al.*, 1998). Chapter 10 considers in more depth the issues involved in calculating and prioritising the cost of aspects of healthcare in relation to clinical guidelines and care protocols. Although in evidence-based practice cost is not usually as overwhelming a consideration as the place that I give it in booking flights, or a buggy, it is still a part of the evidence nonetheless.

Evidence-based practice therefore differs from applying research to practice, because it intends to take a broader view of evidence, to make the practical application of evidence explicit and to acknowledge the individuality of each clinical situation and patient. It includes using information from a variety of sources and requires a critical appraisal of the available evidence, and the appropriate contextual application of this in a real-world situation. It aims to assist practitioners to move beyond routine or ritual care, but its intention is not to replace this with unquestioning acceptance of research or any other form of evidence. It also requires decisions to be made as to whether an intervention can be justified as a cost-effective use of resources.

The concept of evidence-based practice appears a logical way to ensure that a high standard of care is provided. There are, nonetheless, a variety of reasons why it is currently a popular professional, public and political issue. There are three broad subdivisions of groups concerned with the drive to evidence-based practice: professional concerns, public concerns and political concerns. While these groups have many things in common in their quest for quality of care, the agendas of each group, and the priorities which they have, may differ.

THE DEVELOPMENT OF EVIDENCE-BASED PRACTICE

The current drive to engage in evidence-based practice arises from contemporary issues in healthcare, but it is not a new concept, having been discussed as early as 1900 (Sackett *et al.*, 1996). Although the term, 'evidence-based practice' is widely used across healthcare professions, it is generally accepted as being derived from the evidence-based medicine movement (Witkin and Harrison, 2001). This is likely to have influenced the dominant types of evidence which are used, as will be discussed in Chapter 2. Although the concepts behind evidence-based practice have therefore existed for many years, the term evidence-based practice has recently become a popular buzz word in healthcare.

Providing quality care is a requirement for individual professionals, and ensuring that their members practise to an acceptable manner is a function of the governing bodies of professions, such as the General Medical Council (GMC) and the Nursing and Midwifery Council (NMC). Concerns over standards of healthcare include the standard of care provided by individual practitioners, standards achieved by organisations such as NHS Trusts and the standards with which professions as a whole are associated. Assurances that the National Health Service and the professions and individual practitioners therein provide quality care are also obviously important for the general public, the recipients of this care and, through taxation, those who fund it. Politically, healthcare is a major part of public spending and an important electoral issue. Demonstrating a commitment to ensuring quality in healthcare is therefore an aim of most political parties.

Political and professional desires to demonstrate to the public that high standards of care are achieved and the best available care given have contributed to the current emphasis on evidence-based practice. There have been well-publicised cases where the standard of care provided or interventions given were not of the highest or even acceptable quality, such as the events which led to the Bristol Inquiry (Kennedy, 2001). This has meant steps needing to be taken to attempt to reassure the public that the safety of patients and the provision of high-quality care are priorities for professionals and the government. There may also have been a need for mechanisms to be put in place to assist professionals to assure themselves that they are providing the highest possible standards of care.

The Bristol Inquiry (Kennedy, 2001) is commonly cited as one of the major events associated with the development of national clinical guidelines in England. The report from this inquiry relates to practices in paediatric cardiac surgery at the Bristol Royal Infirmary between 1984 and 1995, where the mortality of infants under the age of one year having complex cardiac surgery was found to be unacceptably high. Problems with the surgical techniques used, medical and surgical postoperative care, communication between staff and between staff and families were identified in the report. It was suggested that staff felt unable to report concerns about standards of care either due to fear of reprisals or because there was a lack of clarity over reporting pathways. Where concerns were voiced, the procedures to be followed were not clear, and there was found to be an absence of strong clinical leadership. The inquiry into the events at Bristol made 198 recommendations, some of which have been linked to the subsequent focus on evidence-based practice, the development of national standards overseen by NICE and the auditing processes associated with clinical governance. The events of Bristol are therefore associated with a drive to treatment and care being based on demonstrable evidence of efficacy, the development of national standards and national clinical guidelines. Although ongoing government policy has developed the move towards using care protocols and clinical guidelines further (DoH, 2002), the impetus for this is significantly associated with a need to take steps, and for professions and the government to be seen to be taking steps, towards preventing 'another Bristol'.

This need for concrete evidence that the 'best' care is being provided influences the things which are chosen as quality indicators and the type of evidence which is used to demonstrate quality. For example, it is easier to identify and record whether targets for waiting times are achieved than to demonstrate whether staff are respectful to patients. Quality indicators may therefore tend towards the technical or procedural aspects of care, rather than its humanistic elements, even though these may not reflect what patients see as the most important aspects of quality in care provision. The quest by professionals and politicians to demonstrate quality of care is likely to predispose all concerned towards visible, and thus often measurable, evidence that the 'right' care was given, how 'good' that care was and 'proof' of its efficacy. While this may be necessary and reassuring for professionals, politicians and the public, it may mean that important, but unmeasurable, elements of care are omitted from any evaluation of its quality.

PROFESSIONAL CONCERNS

Evidence-based practice is currently seen as a highly desirable goal for all healthcare professions (Plouffe and Seniuk, 2004). The term evidence-based practice is sometimes used as if it were an optional extra, to be included in care when time allows, or viewed as a pinnacle of best practice to be achieved if possible. However, providing care which is based on the current best evidence is not an optional extra for healthcare staff. Nurses and midwives are required to provide care which is based on the best available evidence (NMC, 2002). The guidance that the GMC provides on the duties of a doctor includes keeping their knowledge up to date, respecting patients' views and involving them in decision-making (GMC, 2005). Thus, healthcare professionals who fail to act upon the current best evidence or to involve patients in decision-making so as to identify the best course of action for individuals may be seen as failing to fulfil their basic duties. Chapter 8 discusses the legal and ethical aspects of using clinical guidelines and care protocols, but using the current best available evidence to inform care, and respecting and incorporating the views and preferences of patients in care provision, is not an add-on which healthcare staff can use if they have the time and inclination. It is a requirement.

Healthcare professionals are also required to fulfil the ethical principles of doing good and doing no harm to their patients. The majority of healthcare professionals are well intentioned, and – with some, often notable, exceptions, such as Beverly Allitt (Clothier, 1994) and Harold Shipman (Smith, 2005) – intend to fulfil these obligations. However, good intentions may not be enough to ensure good care. The report into the events of Bristol (Kennedy, 2001) acknowledges that those involved were not bad people and that there was no evidence of deliberate harm being caused to the children there. In many cases individuals nonetheless fell short of providing an acceptable standard of care, and the organisation for which they worked did not facilitate adequate standards being achieved in this instance. Thus, good intentions, or beliefs by individuals that they are doing the best thing, may not be enough to ensure that good or even safe care is provided.

Concerns over standards of care arising from the Bristol Inquiry (Kennedy, 2001) and Shipman Inquiry (Smith, 2005) have been accompanied by other more general concerns over standards, such as the prevalence of hospital-acquired infection, and staff shortages. The overall picture of healthcare is sometimes that of a service struggling to meet the demands placed on it, with compromises often having to be made in relation to the quality of care. Showing that care is based on the current best evidence may provide a means by which professionals can demonstrate that they employ approaches to care that are deemed to be appropriate or which meet basic quality standards. This may be one way of reassuring the public and politicians that, despite adverse publicity, they are doing a good job.

PUBLIC PERCEPTIONS

High-profile cases of individual professional misconduct such as Beverly Allitt's and Harold Shipman's and institutional failings such as the cases associated with paediatric cardiac surgery at Bristol may have decreased public confidence in healthcare. This is not necessarily the case, as polls of the public post Bristol and Shipman showed that there was no overall loss of confidence in healthcare professionals (Hall, 2001). However, the public may require, or benefit from, reassurances regarding the standards of care that they are likely to receive should they become unwell.

There is also a suggestion that the public are keener now than in the past to know why certain treatment or care is or is not recommended. In the past, patients often accepted a view simply because it was expressed by a medical practitioner, but it is now less likely that this will be the case. The improved availability of health-related information means that the public now have more tools with which to question professionals. In addition, changes in society mean that unquestioning deference is no longer given to professionals, including health professionals. There are also a greater number of choices which individuals can make regarding how they manage their health, for example alternative therapies, which may mean that the public are more likely to want to know the success of conventional, in comparison to alternative, medicine.

These combined factors mean that the public are inclined to demand more information and clearer evidence than before that the decisions of professionals are correct, or the right thing for them. There is therefore likely to be a public demand for what could be termed evidence-based practice. As the views of the public influence their voting behaviour, this will influence political enthusiasm for evidence-based practice.

POLITICAL ASPECTS OF EVIDENCE-BASED PRACTICE

There are political imperatives in the current drive towards evidence-based practice, which will be discussed in more detail in Chapter 11. However, a significant part of government policy and a factor which influences the public's voting behaviour is healthcare provision. Healthcare in the United Kingdom is free at the point of delivery, but is publicly funded. Thus, governments must demonstrate to the public that they are committed to using public money wisely and to achieving as high a standard of healthcare as possible. Concerns over the standards of care that patients receive from individual practitioners or organisations are therefore something on which the government must be seen to act.

In addition, there has been a suggestion that the standard of care provided to, or the options for treatment or care available for, individuals varies greatly depending on their place of residence and local priorities. This apparent inequality in healthcare has led to the government seeking to demonstrate that they are committed to achieving greater equity of healthcare provision (DoH, 1998). The concerns over standards of care and equality of provision have led to moves to provide national guidance on what is thought to be best practice and the best use of resources, and to centrally organised monitoring of standards of care provision (DoH, 1998).

Although the professional and political aspects of evidence-based practice both include the aim of providing the best quality of care, politically, there is also a need to demonstrate that there is national equity of provision and that care provision is cost-effective. In later chapters, cost and the political aspects of clinical guidelines and care protocols will be discussed in greater depth. However, it is relevant to note from the outset that, although evidence-based practice involves the appraisal of evidence to inform direct patient care, the milieu in which it has been popularised means that it cannot be separated from the aim to achieve cost-effectiveness and a greater standardisation of care.

Major players in the move towards the development and achievement of national standards of evidence-based healthcare are the National Institute for Clinical Excellence (NICE) in England and Wales and the Scottish Intercollegiate Guidelines Network (SIGN) in Scotland.

NICE AND SIGN

The report from the Bristol Inquiry recommended that one body should be responsible for coordinating all action in England and Wales related to the setting, issuing and keeping under review of national clinical standards and that this should be NICE. NICE was established as a special health authority in England and Wales with the remit of providing the NHS with guidance, based on an evaluation of the evidence of their clinical efficacy and cost-effectiveness, on new and established treatments and technologies (Goodman, 2000). In April 2005, NICE was renamed the National Institute for Health and Clinical Excellence (still abbreviated to NICE) as it took on the functions of the Health Development Agency. The aim of NICE having this additional role was to create a single excellence-in-practice organisation. NICE are now responsible for providing national guidance on the promotion of good health and the prevention and treatment of ill health. NICE are politically independent, but have a role as a national policy-making body whose responsibility is wider and more detached than the consideration of individual patients or healthcare providers (Wailoo *et al.*, 2004). The intention is therefore for NICE to be independent of government but to have the authority necessary to issue national guidance with the expectation that it will be adhered to. NICE currently issue three types of guidance:

- guidance on public health – the promotion of good health and the prevention of ill health;
- guidance on health technologies – the use of new and existing medicines, treatments and procedures;
- guidance on clinical practice – guidance on the appropriate treatment and care of people with specific diseases and conditions.

Currently, NICE produce guidance in three forms:

- technology appraisals, which give guidance on the use of new and existing medicines and treatments, for example NICE have issued guidance on implantable cardioverter defibrillators (NICE, 2000), and the use of drotrecogin for severe sepsis (NICE, 2004a);
- clinical guidelines, which give guidance on the appropriate treatment and care of people with specific diseases and conditions, for example NICE have issued guidance on chronic heart failure (NICE, 2003a), dyspepsia (NICE, 2004b), antenatal care (NICE, 2003d) and self-harm (NICE 2004c);
- guidance on interventional procedures, in which guidance is given on whether a procedure used for diagnosis or treatment is safe enough and works well enough for routine use. An interventional procedure is defined by NICE as a procedure used for diagnosis or treatment that involves one of: making an incision in the patient, gaining access to a bodily cavity without incision, for example by endoscopy, using electromagnetic radiation such as X-rays, lasers or ultraviolet light. For example, NICE have issued guidance on pancreatic islet cell transplantation (NICE, 2003b) and microwave endometrial ablation (NICE, 2003c).

NICE are therefore charged with providing a variety of evidence-based resources, but although issuing national clinical guidelines is within NICE's remit, it is a part, not the entirety, of the organisation's work. NICE do not issue care protocols; however, the evidence that they produce may be used in developing care protocols.

NICE's aim is to provide NHS care professionals with guidance covering all significant areas of morbidity and mortality encountered in the UK (NICE, 2005b). This is a major undertaking, and within NICE six National Collaborating Centres (NCCs) have been established to increase the range of guidance that can be given and thus facilitate the achievement of this aim. Currently, the NCCs are:

- National Collaborating Centre for Acute Care
- National Collaborating Centre for Cancer
- National Collaborating Centre for Chronic Conditions
- National Collaborating Centre for Mental Health
- National Collaborating Centre for Nursing and Supportive Care

- National Collaborating Centre for Primary Care
- National Collaborating Centre for Women's and Children's Health.

In Scotland, national clinical guidelines are developed by the Scottish Inter-collegiate Guideline Network (SIGN). SIGN was formed in 1993 to develop and disseminate national, evidence-based, clinical guidelines, with the intention of improving the effectiveness of healthcare and reducing variations in practice. However, unlike NICE, SIGN was established before the concerns arising from the Bristol Inquiry or similar concerns.

SIGN and NICE therefore both have a remit to develop national, evidence-based guidance in order to improve standards of care and consistency of practice. SIGN and NICE collaborate as far as is possible in their work so as to avoid unnecessary duplication and so that their guideline development programmes complement each other (SIGN, 2005). SIGN and NICE are both members of the Appraisal of Guidelines, Research and Evaluation (AGREE) collaboration. AGREE is an international network of guideline development and appraisal programmes that has produced standards for the development and evaluation of guidelines. All guidelines that are developed according to the AGREE principles should therefore adhere to certain basic standards, which will be discussed in Chapter 5.

SUMMARY

Evidence-based practice is linked with clinical guidelines and care protocols in that these should be developed from an evaluation of the current best evidence of clinical efficacy and cost-effectiveness. Evidence-based practice involves using the evidence from across a range of sources to inform the care of individual patients, taking into account their specific preferences, needs and circumstances. Although evidence-based practice incorporates research, it requires all the relevant research on a subject to be identified and evaluated, and for this to be made clinically applicable. As its name suggests, the focus of evidence-based practice is that the evidence of clinical efficacy and cost-effectiveness must be used in practice, not remain an ideal that never moves beyond the pages of journals or reports. It therefore requires the practical application of evidence to be clear and for practitioners to make decisions regarding how far general recommendations apply in specific cases.

The concept of evidence-based practice is not new, but in England it has become popular in light of concerns over practice being based on tradition or habit rather than evidence of efficacy, highlighted by specific cases of poor practice. There are public, professional and political imperatives which have influenced its current popularisation. Although all parties may share similar concerns about healthcare, based upon evidence of its effectiveness, they may prioritise those concerns differently and for a variety of reasons. An individual patient may focus primarily on knowing that they are receiving the best care, a practitioner may focus primarily on knowing that they are providing the best care to a group of patients, or to patients within their specialist field, while the government may focus on being seen to encourage all professionals to provide a high but equal standard of care to everyone in the country.

A considerable volume of information is available to healthcare staff and the public. This means that clinical guidelines or care protocols, which provide summaries of the current best evidence and how this relates to practice, may be useful to practitioners. NICE has been established as a special health authority in England and Wales to provide advice, based on the evidence of clinical efficacy and cost-effectiveness, on the best use of NHS resources. SIGN serves a similar function in Scotland. Although NICE and SIGN are not affiliated to any political party and act independently of government, their remit is to consider the best overall use of resources as well as the clinical benefits of specific aspects of healthcare. Both develop guidance which is intended to meet the AGREE collaboration standards. From the existence of a collaboration such as AGREE, it is clear that, although national clinical guidelines have developed in England in part in response to cases of poor performance, there is an international as well as national increase in the use of clinical guidelines and an acknowledgement that the guideline development and evaluation process itself should be subject to quality-control mechanisms. Using evidence to inform practice will only contribute to a high quality of care if the evidence itself is of high quality and used in appropriate situations.

2

Evidence

Clinical guidelines and care protocols should be based on the current best evidence of clinical efficacy and cost-effectiveness. In order to develop or effectively use clinical guidelines or care protocols, a knowledge of what constitutes evidence is therefore needed (Heitkemper and Bond, 2004). Isolated pieces of evidence can be misleading, and as well as understanding what is considered to contribute to evidence, knowing how to weigh up all the evidence is necessary.

Some of my friends and colleagues tend to express concern when I head towards South America. They seem to think, or maybe hope, that I will become a victim of violent crime and that they will never see me again. On my last trip, my backpack was stolen in Chile. This was enough evidence for some of the prophets of doom to consider their point proven, and so I supposedly had to put up with those annoying 'I told you so' facial expressions and tilts of the head (which aren't actually evidence of sympathy but mean that they really think it serves you right for not listening to them in the first place). Galvanised by those very looks, I remain stubbornly unconvinced. Admittedly, I have had a backpack stolen in South America. I have also had a backpack stolen from a locker at the Royal Brompton Hospital's paediatric intensive care unit (PICU), a mobile phone and wallet stolen on Waterloo Station, a camera stolen in Brighton, a massive credit card fraud in Sheffield, my car broken into in the same city, a bike stolen from Addenbrooke's Hospital and another from Charing Cross Hospital. The most irritating crime of all and the one whose perpetrator I would most like to slap was having the straps from my infant bike seat stolen at Southampton Central Railway Station. The seat was left there, to remind me of what I had in mind for an armful of seven-month-old baby and a bike, but the straps were taken, so that when I reached that happy point of being almost home from work I had no way of actually getting myself and my baby the last two miles. That was very annoying indeed and may have resulted in young John learning immoderate language. So, the evidence is there, for those who want it, that there are thieves in South America, and that they may nick your stuff. However, it should perhaps be balanced with the evidence of crime in England and the many times when I have been in South

America and experienced no crime at all. For interest's sake, I also had a T-shirt stolen in Te Anau, New Zealand, and my partner had his boxer shorts stolen from a washing machine in Australia's capital city.

The aim of evidence-based practice according to Sackett *et al.* (1996) and Di Censo *et al.* (1998) is to use the best evidence from all the available sources to form a balanced judgement. This includes using the findings from research, but, as was described in Chapter 1, evidence-based practice differs from simply finding what seems to be relevant research and then using this in practice settings. It requires research and other forms of evidence to be evaluated and synthesised so that a composite picture of the current best evidence is obtained. This is then applied to real-world practice by deciding what is the best course of action in relation to a particular aspect of healthcare practice. Finally, evidence-based practice requires practitioners to use their clinical expertise in conjunction with patient preference to decide how appropriate such recommendations are in each specific care setting and for each individual patient.

This chapter discusses what is meant by evidence in the context of evidence-based practice, the sources of evidence which are likely to be used, how the relative value which will be attributed to different types of evidence is decided and how decisions are made as to what evidence to use.

WHAT IS EVIDENCE?

Before discussing the sources of evidence that may be used in evidence-based practice, it is useful to discuss what evidence is. The *Oxford English Dictionary* (2001) defines 'evidence' as 'Information or signs indicating whether a belief or proposition is true or valid' and: 'Information used to establish facts.'

Evidence-based practice therefore requires the gathering of information related to an aspect of care to determine whether what is believed or proposed to be best practice actually is.

Seeking information which represents the facts may not be as easy as it seems, as what is considered to be a 'fact' varies. How a physicist perceives 'fact' will be very different from 'fact' as seen by a psychologist. The 'facts' which healthcare professionals perceive to be relevant to patient care may be very different from the 'facts' which patients see as important. For example a physician may measure how effective interventions are in terms of physiological measurements. However, patients may view how well their disease is controlled in terms of the limitations placed on their life. If they have to reduce their work hours and social life and take medications which have significant side effects in order to achieve a reduction in symptoms, they may see their disease as poorly controlled, despite an improvement in physiological variables. Thus, the physician may see the 'fact' as being that the prescribed medical interventions and alterations in lifestyle have effectively controlled the disease process and improved the patient's health. The patient, on the other hand, may see the 'fact' as being that the interventions are ineffective as they still have a poor quality of life overall despite these.

This example illustrates that, although evidence is based on finding facts, there are different types of facts, for example the measurable fact that a blood result is improved, the less easily measurable fact that a patient has had to alter their work hours and commitments and goals to achieve a reduction of symptoms and the unmeasurable fact that a woman feels that she cannot offer her child as much attention or assistance with out-of-school activities as other parents can because of her illness. All of these facts are important in determining what is best for the individual, and, because the nature of these facts differs, the optimum way to find out about and present them also differs.

There are a range of ways in which evidence which contributes to our understanding of healthcare can be explored and presented. The Cochrane Collaboration (2004) and Centre for Reviews and Dissemination (CRD) (2001) describe evidence as including the findings from research, expert opinion, papers based on physiological principles, consensus view, cost, patient preference, and practitioner's expertise in the evidence which should inform practice. Given this range of sources of evidence, and the need to make decisions about what should be recommended in practice, the relative weight that will be attached to each type of evidence in any situation must be decided. Evidence is therefore usually arranged in what are termed hierarchies of evidence. These show how important each form of evidence is considered to be in comparison with other forms of evidence. Although there is more to evidence-based practice than applying research findings, research is usually seen as the highest form of evidence.

RESEARCH

Research is defined as: 'The systematic study of materials and sources in order to establish facts and reach new conclusions' (Oxford English Dictionary, 2001).

Research should involve systematically and rigorously gathering evidence on a given subject. Because it uses systematic and rigorous processes, the information generated using research is considered likely to be a more accurate representation of fact than other forms of evidence (CRD, 2001). Because of this, it is usually seen as a high-quality form of evidence, and given the highest place in hierarchies of evidence (Harbour and Miller, 2001).

Although research is usually described as the highest form of evidence, there are a range of ways in which research can be conducted. The research methods used depend upon the type of information being sought. The overarching way in which research is conducted is often described as being divided into paradigms, or methodologies. The methodology or paradigm that is most appropriate to find information about a subject depends upon what is being investigated, how knowledge will be generated or the beliefs about what knowledge is which underpin the investigation. What distinguishes research in general from more casual investigation is that it should be detailed and systematic and follow the rules or beliefs of the paradigm to which it is affiliated and comply with the ethical principles which underpin research.

Two major subdivisions of research which are often alluded to in healthcare are positivist and naturalistic, or quantitative and qualitative, inquiry.

Positivist/Quantitative Inquiry

The traditional focus of knowledge generation in healthcare, and particularly in medicine, has been positivist (or quantitative) research. In positivist research in healthcare, establishing cause and effect is usually the object, and the methods used to investigate interventions and their effectiveness aim to demonstrate how confidently it can be assumed that a given action produces a certain result. Although casual observation might seem to show cause and effect, this is not always the case.

In Alberta, somewhere on the road from Jasper to Lake Louise, our Greyhound Bus was involved in a Bear Jam Collision. A black bear had put in an appearance at the roadside. All the traffic slowed, to look at the bear, take photos and videos. All, that is, except the RV behind us, which hit us with enough force to fling its woman passenger, who had been standing up at the front of the vehicle, through the windscreen. A short interval of rescue, first aid and ghoulish videoing by those who were so inclined ensued. Then everyone stood around waiting for the helicopter to take the casualty back to Calgary. At this point, the bear reappeared, wandering demurely by the roadside, wondering what all the fuss was about. One of our copassengers, who had shown an unhealthy interest in videoing the woman while she was under the RV and was now rather at a loose end, turned his video bearwards: 'This is the bear that caused the accident,' he confided into his microphone.

This seemed a little harsh. After all, the bear wasn't really responsible – he was just going about his bear-like business at the roadside. The cause of the accident was, I would guess, composed of a number of factors: the fact that the woman was standing up at the front of an RV, the fact that her husband didn't keep an eye on what the other traffic was doing and the fact that a bear appeared to distract everyone's attention from boring things like road safety. The bear wasn't the absolute cause, because there were plenty of other vehicles that did not fling their passengers through the window at the sight of a bear. Thus, the suggestion of cause and effect being the bear and an accident were not, in my opinion, quite accurate or fair on the bear. And the fact that

I was irritated by the accident-spotting video operator added to my feeling of injustice on the part of the bear.

In healthcare, showing cause and effect is often a little more important. The bear is probably not really concerned that he has been accused, perhaps somewhat harshly, of causing accidents and will doubtless continue to wander the roadsides unperturbed. However, the confidence with which it can be assumed that administering a certain drug at a given dose will provide pain relief without excessive side effects is rather more important. Because the intention is to provide evidence of cause and effect (for example that giving a drug will have the effect of producing pain relief) which can be used with confidence, widely generalisable facts are sought in positivist inquiry (Greenhalgh, 1999). The safety and effectiveness of therapeutic interventions must therefore be tested in a manner that allows their widespread and confident use. One of the main approaches to this type of knowledge generation is the randomised controlled trial (RCT).

Positivist research relies on measurable data and numerical facts, with the quest being to produce evidence that is statistically significant so that the findings can be confidently applied across entire populations. To this end, large numbers of participants or research subjects are involved. The selection of research subjects and how the research is conducted must also minimise the effects of variables which might confound the findings: these are factors which might cause the findings to appear to be due to an intervention when in fact they are not or which might cause the intervention to appear ineffective when in fact it is. In the case of the bear, it was assumed that he was the cause, but there were contributory factors, such as the injured party being engaged in some activity at the front of the RV and that the RV's driver did not slow or stop his vehicle when everyone else did (which could have been the distraction of the dancing woman beside him but could also have been that he was drunk, on drugs or some other cause of poor concentration). In research respecting the effect of a drug, this might include coexisting diagnoses which could affect the physiological variables being used as measures of the drug's effectiveness. These are not a part of the disease for which the drug is being tested; so, although they may affect the perceived effectiveness of the drug, they would detract from, or confound, what is actually being investigated.

Attempts can be made to reduce this type of variable, for example by excluding individuals with known coexisting diagnoses or health problems. However, not all variables will be known or be able to be controlled. For example, not all patients with a given disease will have had this diagnosed or disclose it to researchers. In the case of the bear, if we assume that the RV not stopping was affected by either the bear, the antics of the driver's wife/partner/hitchhiker distracting him or poor driving skills from some other cause, research concerning the actual cause would need to address how far dancing women, the bear and poor driving skills contributed to this. However, there might be other variables within this, such as whether the driver liked the woman or her front-of-RV activities and how much this, rather than just her presence at the front of the vehicle or the bear being beside the roadside, contributed. These might be difficult to elicit. It is therefore also necessary to conduct positivist research in such a way that unknown or unpredictable factors are unlikely to significantly influence the results. One method of achieving this is by having a sufficiently large sample size that the effects of some participants having such variables would not affect the overall study results. For example, if a sample of 10 000 RV drivers in Canada was used, the effect of one of them secretly wanting to flick his wife out of the window to a black bear would affect study results much less significantly than in a sample of ten.

One further method used to ensue that, within the sample involved in the research, there is no difference between those receiving an intervention and those not doing so, or an equal chance of each group having unknown variables which might affect the intervention, is randomisation. In randomisation, within what is considered to be a homogeneous group, one group is allocated one intervention, such as a new drug, and another is allocated either no intervention or an intervention with which the first is being compared. The selection of which individual is allocated to each group is completely random. For example, in an RCT of the use of inhaled versus intravenous steroids in treating acute asthma, a large group of participants would be recruited and, although half of the group would receive each intervention, there would be an equal chance of each individual receiving inhaled or injected steroids. In the bear and RV scenario, if we assume that the RV not stopping was affected by either the bear, the antics of the woman or poor driving, a large sample of drivers could be made to drive into a traffic jam, some going past bears, some with women dancing at the front of their RV and some without any distraction. The way in which each driver was allocated to each group would be completely random so that factors such as them disliking their wife would not influence which group they were placed in. There would then be an equal chance of everyone being placed in the 'dancing wives' group, and of those in the group liking their wives as not.

A controlled trial is one in which there is a group that receives an intervention and a group that does not. Those receiving the intervention under investigation are the experimental group, and those not receiving the intervention under investigation are the control group. This might mean one group receiving a new intervention and one receiving an established intervention or might mean one group receiving an intervention and one receiving no intervention. Controlling should allow a judgement to be made as to whether any effect which is observed is due to the intervention or whether it simply reflects the number of patients who would always have, for example, died, recovered or improved. If an intervention is given to an entire group, with no control group against which to compare it, inferring that any change in condition is due to the intervention is less reasonable, as the fate of those not receiving the intervention is unknown. For example, in the case of our friend the bear, an RCT to see if the bear really was the cause would involve two groups: one group, the control group, would be men driving old RVs through Canada with a dancing woman at the front, the experimental group would do the same, but with a bear appearing by the roadside. That way, although the dancing woman and driving skills might contribute to the accident, whether the bear really made the chances of an accident higher or not could be shown. In this case, the research would then need to have groups with just the driver, the driver with a dancing woman and the driver with a dancing woman and a bear at the roadside, to see if a combination of events was more likely to produce the accident. If the same number of accidents happened when men were driving with no distraction as when they had the combined forces of a dancer and a bear, it might mean that the woman and the bear were irrelevant: accidents just happen now and then. It would be a complex study, needs a little more refinement and is not my usual area of specialism, but, for a year or so in Canada, I would be prepared to do it.

The aim of an RCT is therefore to reduce the likelihood of what seem to be the findings from research being purely a result of chance and not an outcome of an intervention. The intention is therefore to increase the confidence with which any effect, positive or negative, can be attributed to the intervention in question.

'Blinding' is another term that is commonly used in positivist research. Here, the research subjects do not know whether they are in the experimental or control group of the research. For example, in a blind RCT of a new drug which is being used to treat cancer, patients who have agreed to be in the trial would not know if they were receiving the new drug or established treatment. Blinding aims to reduce the potential bias that might arise from an individual knowing that they have, or have not, received a given intervention. For example, in a trial of analgesics, because of the complexities of pain perception and reporting, knowing whether or not they have received a trial drug might affect an individual's perception and reporting of pain. Although blinding may be useful, it is not always possible. For example, if one group of patients were receiving reflexology and one were not, it would not be possible to blind participants to whether or not they were experiencing the use of reflexology. However, in a drug trial, it is often possible to use blinding. The bear study would not really be suitable for blinding, as the driver would be bound to know if there was a woman dancing at the front of his RV or not. If he didn't, that might point to the cause.

In some circumstances, it is also possible and appropriate to use what is known as 'double blinding', in which neither the research subject nor those providing the intervention know whether an individual is in the intervention or control group. For example, in a double-blind trial a nurse who is administering the drugs involved will not know if they were actually administering a trial drug or a placebo. There will always be a record of which participants receive each intervention, but in a double-blind trial those who are directly involved in giving or receiving the intervention do not know this.

The 'gold standard' tool in positivist research, in which the greatest chance of ascertaining whether any findings are due to the intervention in question and not other factors and from which findings can most confidently be applied would therefore be a double-blind RCT. However, this approach is not always possible. Neither does a study being described as a double-blind RCT guarantee that it is of high quality. A double-blind RCT may be badly designed, produce poor data or reach conclusions that are not valid. It may use insufficient numbers to generate findings that are of statistical significance, the statistical analysis may be performed incorrectly or the study may be conducted in a manner which is not rigorous or which is biased. Thus, when evidence is being sought and evaluated, although an RCT is often cited as the highest form of evidence, each RCT is only as good as the study itself. It is also only a valid way of generating evidence if the subject being investigated is appropriate for the use of positivist/quantitative methodology and an RCT. Using an RCT to investigate a subject which is not appropriate for this type of inquiry will not produce good evidence.

Naturalistic Research

Although positivist research is the means by which medical knowledge has traditionally been generated, this approach is not appropriate for seeking facts about all aspects of healthcare. Health and therefore healthcare consists of more than quantifiable facts. It includes individual perceptions, values and priorities, beliefs about health and illness, and the effects of health on individuals' lives (Witkin and Harrison, 2001; Mulhall *et al.*, 2001). The efficacy of various drugs and other therapeutic approaches to treating Alzheimer's disease may be evaluated using RCTs, but understanding the concerns of the families of people with Alzheimer's disease cannot be investigated effectively using RCTs. Measurable facts relating to any given condition or disease process may exist, but the context in which these occur and the complex biopsychosocial elements of health and illness involve specific problems or issues for individual patients and their families (Weissman, 2000). This may include the effect that their illness has on their quality of life, how they perceive themselves as a result of their illness and their views on the way in which healthcare professionals treat them. As these are not measurable facts, gathering information by using quantitative (positivist) research, which uses numerical measures, will be inappropriate. For example, it would be difficult to measure how patients with motor neurone disease made decisions regarding their long-term care. It might be possible to measure how many individuals who are diagnosed with this condition and who are involved in the healthcare services are cared for at home and how many are cared for in residential accommodation or hospital. However, understanding how these decisions are reached and how satisfied patients and their families are with the available options is less easy to evaluate numerically. Numerical evaluation is also unlikely to enhance an understanding of the complexities of decision-making and satisfaction therewith for patients and their families.

A recognition of the multifaceted nature of health and healthcare and the inadequacy of numerical evaluation for understanding all aspects of it has led to an increasing acceptance of methods of inquiry other than positivism. This often means using qualitative, or naturalistic, methodologies.

Naturalistic approaches to knowledge generation seek to explore the understanding of a situation and the meanings and values attributed to this by individuals, rather than seeking numerical proof of facts that can then be generalised across wide populations. Their focus is not to prove cause and effect in the way that positivist inquiry does. For example, mortality amongst neonates who undergo high-frequency oscillation ventilation for respiratory distress syndrome compared to those who do not can be measured statistically. However, there will also be issues for the families of these infants that cannot be accurately portrayed using statistical measures. It may be possible to develop statistical evidence about broad areas of concern which parents have, such as: that their baby will die, have significant residual health problems or disability and the loss of their expected transition to parenting. However, the depth and nature of these concerns, and the ways in which families perceive care and their dealings with healthcare staff, cannot be reduced to statistical measurements. Neither can such experiences necessarily be neatly generalised across populations. While it is probably true to state that all parents of neonates who require high-frequency oscillation ventilation are likely to be concerned that their baby may die, their priorities in terms of sustaining life at any cost, their coping mechanisms and the ways in which they should be supported during this time cannot be prescribed in the way that a drug dose and route of administration can. The aim of naturalistic inquiry in this situation is to help healthcare staff to understand what this situation is like for families and what their experiences are, and thus enable them to provide better care.

Rather than attempting to control variables and to render the context of individual research subjects unimportant, so that it can be assumed that the findings apply to everyone in a given situation, in qualitative research, context is all-important. In quantitative research, the precise circumstances of each research subject should not be an issue as the aim is to achieve a homogeneous sample and to demonstrate whether an intervention will be effective across an entire population. In contrast, in qualitative inquiry, a detailed understanding of each individual's potentially idiosyncratic circumstances is essential as this methodology acknowledges and emphasises the individuality of each person's experience. Qualitative research reports should therefore include contextual details that will allow judgements to be made by those using the research regarding its applicability to their own practice.

In qualitative inquiry, sample size is smaller than in quantitative research in order to allow the necessary depth of exploration to take place. As there is no quest for statistical significance or to achieve generalisability, sample sizes do not need to be large enough to control variables. Because depth of information is sought, large sample sizes, instead of enhancing a study's quality, might detract from the quality of the inquiry by preventing an adequate depth of exploration from being achieved. Randomisation, controlling and blinding are also not typically used in qualitative research. In most cases, this would be inappropriate or impossible.

There are a vast range of methods of naturalistic inquiry, dependent upon what is being investigated and why. There is no one best method of naturalistic inquiry akin to positivist RCTs. What is always essential is to determine what is being investigated and whether the methods being used are appropriate for this.

THE BEST METHOD OF RESEARCH

Both positivist and naturalistic inquiry have an important place in healthcare research and therefore in generating evidence to inform practice (Mulhall, 1998). Neither is innately superior, and their worth is related to how appropriately they are used and the quality of individual pieces of research. For example, naturalistic inquiry would be of limited value for exploring the effectiveness of techniques used for cardiac surgery. However, it would be appropriate for exploring the information needs of parents whose child had undergone cardiac surgery. Positivist inquiry and in particular an RCT would be appropriate in the former case and of limited value in the latter. In some cases, a subject may merit both positivist and naturalistic inquiry and use mixed methods of data collection and analysis to explore both qualitative and quantitative aspects of a given healthcare situation. For example, if a new drug is being tested, quantitative research would be used to test its safety and efficacy, but qualitative inquiry may be a valuable adjunct to this to explore the factors that influence patient compliance in taking it. Both types of research would be important to ensure as far as is possible that the drug is safe but also to understand whether or not it will be used. Prescribing an extremely effective drug will be of limited value if it is not taken and may be a waste of resources if it is dispensed but not taken.

In all forms of research the quality of the specific study or studies is as important to note as the methodology used. Any study may be methodologically flawed. This includes the wrong paradigm being selected to explore an issue, the researcher selecting inappropriate methods of data collection for the matter being investigated, the analysis process being flawed or the researcher drawing inaccurate conclusions from the data. Studies may also be biased. For example, if they are funded by parties with a vested interest in producing certain findings, pressure may be exerted on the research team to interpret or present results in a way which shows their product in a more favourable light than they should. Funding from pharmaceutical companies is widely cited as particularly problematic as companies generally aim to prove their product to be safe and more effective than alternative drugs on the market. Other possible sources of funding bias nonetheless exist, for example a counselling service funding naturalistic inquiry into the benefit of counselling for post-traumatic stress disorder might be open to such bias.

The way in which research should be evaluated depends upon the type of research being undertaken. As qualitative and quantitative research have different aims and use different methods of data collection and analysis, the same indicators of quality cannot be used for both. Quantitative research aims to identify cause and effect and to control variables in order to allow the data generated to be generalised to a wide population. In contrast, qualitative approaches view the context in which events occur as essential and do not seek to reduce findings to levels of statistical significance. As the intention of each type of research is very different, the criteria used to evaluate a study's quality are also distinct. Evaluating a quantitative study using criteria intended for qualitative research (or vice versa) would not be a good indicator of a study's quality.

The positivist paradigm uses criteria of reliability, validity and generalisability to indicate the quality of research. However, these criteria are not appropriate for use with qualitative inquiry. The criteria used in qualitative research vary according to the exact methodology used, and the beliefs that underpin this. However, it is generally based on whether an adequate depth of inquiry has been conducted, whether the study accurately portrays the truth of a situation and whether systematic processes have been followed.

In evidence-based practice, as well as the quality of each study, the importance that will be attached to each form of evidence must be decided. These decisions allow hierarchies of evidence to be developed in which each type of evidence is graded according to how much weight it will carry in making recommendations. Although 'research' is usually regarded as the best form of evidence, the type of research that this refers to will depend upon the subject in question. How closely each paradigm fits the phenomenon being explored is the crucial point in deciding its place in hierarchies of evidence. For example, although naturalistic research is a form of research, and therefore a high-ranking form of evidence, it would not be appropriate for investigating the effectiveness of a drug being used to treat hypertension. It would therefore not be high in the hierarchy of evidence on this subject. This is not to say that this form of research is not good, just that it is not appropriate in this instance. Similarly, an RCT would not be appropriate for investigating children with cancer's understanding of death and would therefore not be high in a hierarchy of evidence on this subject.

As Chapter 1 identified, evidence-based practice has, traditionally, held a medical bias. Medicine has a strong culture of using positivist research, as its intention has generally been to identify cause and effect in relation to diseases and interventions. Evidence-based practice is influenced by this culture. Witkin and Harrison (2001) and Schulkin (2000) suggest that this has meant that qualitative research is usually placed lower in hierarchies of evidence than positivist inquiry, even when this is not appropriate. In some cases, it will be appropriate for positivist research to hold the higher status. However, this should only occur in situations in which positivist inquiry is the more appropriate approach to knowledge generation, not because inappropriate evaluative criteria are applied to naturalistic inquiry.

Clinical guidelines and care protocols are generally developed with the intention of making widely generalisable recommendations. In the case of recommendations by NICE and SIGN, the intention is to provide national guidance. It is therefore often appropriate that quantitative findings dominate, as this type of inquiry aims to produce generalisable results. This is not to say they are inherently superior, simply that where wide generalisation is sought the quantitative paradigm is usually more appropriate. As well as deciding which type of research or other form of evidence is the most appropriate for exploring any subject, whether the subject is suitable for guideline or protocol development should be considered. Chapter 5 will explore how subjects should be selected for guideline or protocol development. However, there is much more to healthcare than following clinical guidelines or care protocols. If qualitative inquiry is the most appropriate form of evidence regarding a subject, trying to make it fit a tool whose intention is wide generalisability is likely to be inappropriate. There are vital elements of care provision for which developing clinical guidelines or care protocols is inappropriate, and many elements of care which are suitable for qualitative inquiry fall within this category.

SUMMARISING EVIDENCE FROM RESEARCH

Evidence-based practice requires the evidence from all sources to be summarised. In quantitative inquiry, and in particular when RCTs are used, a commonly used way to merge and summarise data across studies is the statistical method known as meta-analysis. This approach effectively increases the sample size being considered by pooling the results from more than one study (Lancaster et al., 1997). For example, it has been used in collating the evidence concerning pre-oxygenation for tracheal suctioning in intubated, ventilated neonates (Pritchard et al., 2002) and the use of antibiotics for preventing respiratory tract infections in adults receiving intensive care (Liberati et al., 2002). By increasing the sample size, meta-analysis allows the confidence with which findings can be attributed to the intervention in question to be increased.

Meta-analysis is the most widely accepted way of synthesising positivist findings and generalising these as far as is possible. There is nonetheless a risk of overgeneralisation of results or pooling of results from studies which were not in fact intended to measure the same phenomenon or which did not use sufficiently similar patient groups or methods to be meaningfully combined. Meta-analysis is not a method of summarising all results across all studies. It should only be used to pool results which are about phenomena and use data-collection methods which are similar enough to allow the valid combining of data. If data are pooled from investigations which use significantly different approaches to data generation, or across studies which do not actually measure the same thing or the same population, the recommendations from the meta-analysis are likely to be unreliable. To return to the accused Canadian black bear, if the aim is to establish if the bear caused the accident, only data from studies of bear jams should be used. It might be tempting to use data from moose jams, particularly if the data from bear jams is limited, but using the findings from moose jams would not be appropriate if the factor being investigated were the bear, not interesting Canadian animals in general.

Meta-analysis is not used in qualitative inquiry, where the reduction of findings to statistical data is inappropriate. One approach to summarising the findings from qualitative studies is metasynthesis. This approach can be used to combine the theories, narratives and interpretations from more than one study by comparing the findings from across studies and integrating these in order to enlarge and broaden an understanding of the phenomenon under investigation (Nelson, 2002). Meta-analysis seeks to merge a variety of statistical data into one data set and thus reduce several studies to one set of numerical findings that will have greater statistical significance and thus wider generalisability. Metasynthesis does not aim to increase generalisability by increasing the sample size, as is the case in meta-analysis. Instead, metasynthesis aims to provide a broader and deeper view (Beck, 2002). The intentions and methods used in meta-analysis and metasynthesis are therefore congruent with their respective paradigms. However, despite assurances that metasynthesis does not aim to reduce data, Thorne *et al.* (2002) suggest that in qualitative inquiry in general there is a tendency to reduce experiences into single overarching themes or patterns so that these can be neatly stated, rather than an attempt to convey their complexity. This applies equally to metasynthesis, where the risk of findings being neatly reduced to succinct themes is perhaps even higher. Where metasynthesis is used, there should be no attempt to make it fit a positivist model. Each approach should be used for appropriate areas of inquiry and for appropriate purposes.

OTHER SOURCES OF EVIDENCE

Research is generally seen as the highest form of evidence. Other sources of knowledge nonetheless can and should contribute to the evidence that informs practice. These include expert opinion, case reports and papers based on physiological principles (CRD, 2001).

Case reports are generally given a lower place in the hierarchy of evidence than research as they usually report only one or two cases, meaning that, from a positivist viewpoint, the points observed cannot be generalised in the way that those encountered in a large RCT can. Despite reporting the findings from a real-world practice situation, case reports have not usually been subjected to the rigorous quality processes which are required for research and are therefore also placed lower in hierarchies of evidence for qualitative inquiry.

Case reports have an important part to play in developing treatment and interventions, particularly in new areas of practice where research has yet to be conducted or where research may not be viable. For example, a new technique for studying cerebral perfusion would probably initially be reported in a case report or reports. This, supported by a discussion of anatomical and physiological principles, may be extremely important in developing a new and potentially useful tool which will improve head-injury management. However, other practitioners would not be able to use this as confidently (because of a lack of knowledge of the likely risks and benefits) as an intervention which had been tested across a large population, and where success had been demonstrated in a statistically significant proportion of cases. It may also be useful in cases where a disease is relatively rare and where it is unlikely that enough cases will be available to conduct quantitative research but where guidance still needs to be developed.

In qualitative inquiry, clarity is needed over the use of the terms 'case report' and 'case study'. The latter can be a form of research (Hewitt-Taylor, 2002), and the former, a case report which has not been subjected to the quality mechanisms of research, is not. For example, a case study of a woman suffering from post-partum depression would expect to use in-depth and rigorous processes of inquiry to explore her experiences, her feelings, her relationships with her baby and family, her experiences of treatment and her interactions with professionals. A case report would probably be briefer and report the presenting symptoms, treatment and interventions given and responses to these.

Papers based on physiological principles are also generally seen as lower forms of evidence than research. Like case reports, these can be useful in generating an evidence base for practice where guidance is needed but empirical work has yet to be carried out, or cannot be carried out. There are instances where an RCT might be desirable, but where it will be problematic, practically or ethically, to conduct one. Thus, despite an RCT being an ideal form of evidence, other ways of making decisions are needed. It may also be that conducting research related to certain interventions in a given client group, for example in children or pregnant women, is problematic. In such situations, the known physiology of childhood or pregnancy may be combined with evidence from research in other population groups to reach conclusions respecting the likely risk of an intervention.

Physiological principles may also be used as adjuncts to expert opinion or case reports to explain why experts prefer certain approaches to treatment or why it is thought that a given intervention produced a given result. Thus, some papers that are used to inform practice may be a combination of types of evidence. Therefore, other types of evidence may not be able to be neatly categorised but are usually seen as lower in the hierarchy of evidence than research.

EXPERT OPINION

Expert opinion is an important part of the evidence that should inform practice (Sackett *et al.*, 1996). However, despite being potentially derived from years of experience, the consensus views of experts have not been subjected to the systematic approach to inquiry which is demanded in research and thus papers based on expert opinion are not usually considered to be as high-ranking a form of evidence as research findings.

Opinion papers written by experts in the field of practice may be combined with physiological principles or a case report. Where there is inadequate research available, the consensus view of a number of experts, drawn from a variety of cases, or their beliefs based on applied physiological principles, is especially useful to enable recommendations to be made. A consensual view, rather than the view of an individual, is preferable as discussion and gaining the perspectives of a number of experts, across all the disciplines involved in an area of practice, make the outcome less likely to be subjective. One of the aims of evidence-based practice is, according to Sackett *et al.* (1996) not to refute expert judgement but rather to develop it and acknowledge this as a valid form of evidence, provided it is expertise, and not uninformed preference, which is being promoted. Having a consensual opinion, backed by physiological principles and applied to a particular case or cases which explain why an intervention is thought to be successful, is preferable to one individual's unsubstantiated opinion becoming accepted practice. Returning to our American bear spotter, the unsubstantiated view of one video-waving bystander on the culpability of the bear is not really enough. However, if a large group of acknowledged experts in the field of road accidents, the effects of bears on driving and the effects that dancing women have on RV drivers came to the conclusion that, despite an absence of empirical evidence, it seemed that bears wandering by roadsides were responsible for causing accidents, and supported this with a range of case studies, in which traffic of various types and with a range of drivers, were adversely affected by bears, this suggestion would carry greater weight.

An example of where expert opinion and a consensual view have been used in developing national guidelines is the Royal College of Nursing's (RCN) guideline on pressure-relieving devices (RCN, 2001). The guideline's development group state that, although evidence from RCTs would have been the ideal form of evidence in this case, where these were not available, other forms of evidence, including the consensual views of experts were used. They make clear that such evidence resulted in recommendations which are not as strong as those derived from RCTs, but that this represents the current best available evidence in an area of practice in which clear guidance is needed (RCN, 2001). Similarly, Aiello *et al.* (2004) also describe the development of a guideline for intravitreous infusion to manage ocular disease where consensus from experienced surgeons and industry representatives was accepted in areas where research on the subject was incomplete or unavailable.

Documents which describe expert opinions and the consensual views of a group of experts are forms of evidence which may be used to develop clinical guidelines and care protocols. However, individual clinical expertise in appropriately applying the composite findings from across a number of sources is also a vital part of evidence-based practice (Sackett *et al.*, 1996; Di Censo *et al.*, 1998). This will be discussed further in Chapter 8, but expertise in practice which enables practitioners to appropriately apply evidence to individual patient situations cannot be placed in a hierarchy of evidence. It is an intrinsic part of care and should be integral to every part of practice.

PATIENT PREFERENCES

NICE (2004j) identify that the views of those who receive healthcare should form a part of the evidence that informs practice. Approaches to placing the views of patients in a hierarchy of evidence is similar to the processes followed for placing expertise in a hierarchy of evidence. Patients' views may be a form of research where there is research that explores patients' perspectives. For example, qualitative research might be used to explore the views of parents whose children have Down syndrome on the antenatal screening and counselling that they received. In this case, the way in which the place of these parents' views in the hierarchy of evidence is determined will be the same as for determining the place of any form of research.

Ascertaining patients' views may also be achieved by using patient groups or societies to identify the consensual view of patients in the same way that the consensual views of experts may be determined. For the same reason, this will usually have a lower place in the hierarchy of evidence than research, because it has not been subjected to the quality mechanisms of research.

As with expert opinion, there are two main facets of patient opinion or preference in evidence-based practice. One is the documentation of patient preference which can be placed in a hierarchy of evidence, according to the type of evidence that it is, as described in the examples above. The second is discovering and acting upon the preferences and views of individual patients. Like expertise in practice being a vital part of every care encounter, consideration of individual patient need and preference is an essential part of every

care situation and cannot be placed in a hierarchy of evidence. It is a requirement of practice on every occasion that a healthcare professional is in contact
with a patient.

COST

As well as considering the relative importance of evidence from research and
other documentary sources, cost-effectiveness is a driving force in healthcare.
In a National Health Service funded by public money but free at the point of
delivery, and in which central resources must be used for the good of all, cost-
effectiveness is a necessary consideration (Goodman, 2000). At national and
local levels decisions made for the care of one patient will impact on the
resources and thus the care available for others.

Cost may be considered as a stand-alone factor, for example the cost of one
drug compared to another and the benefit and cost likely to be derived from
the drug being used. However, cost influences every type of evidence. The cost
of conducting research influences whether or not it can be carried out. Funding
for research must often be gained from outside the NHS, frequently from
private companies, drug companies or companies which manufacture medical
products. Funding can therefore introduce bias and affect the quality of
research. It also means that, even with private funding, some research that
might be beneficial cannot be conducted, owing to insufficient funds being
available. Research being conducted in one area often means that research in
another area cannot be carried out, as funding is only available for one project.
When research is conducted, expert opinion generated or clinical guidelines
or care protocols developed, this involves staff time, which is a costly resource.
The cost of spending time with patients and ascertaining their views,
wishes and preferences is costly and may reduce the time that staff have to
spend on other aspects of care or with other patients. The implementation of
new findings has a cost implication related to the cost of products or equipment that may be needed, staff training and the evaluation of changes in
practice.

Thus, to suggest that cost can be ignored, or is a peripheral part of healthcare, is unrealistic. Evidence-based practice should be immersed in reality and
must therefore include cost as a real part of the factors which inform the recommendations made (Hewitt-Taylor, 2003). Far from considering cost implications as unnecessary or even unethical, the reality is that it is unrealistic and
indeed unethical not to consider the cost and resource implications of a given
course of action. However, the strength of the evidence regarding cost, the relative benefits of an intervention and the strength of other forms of evidence
and the cost over time of non-intervention as well as the cost of intervention
must be considered. Chapter 10 discusses cost issues in relation to clinical
guidelines and care protocols in more depth; however, cost is an issue which

cannot, and should not, be ignored in healthcare in general or in evidence-based practice.

SUMMARY

There are a range of sources that should contribute to the evidence which informs healthcare practice. These include research, expert opinion, case studies, physiological principles, patients' views and cost. The sources of evidence used are generally organised into hierarchies of evidence, to indicate the importance which is attributed to each one and the influence which each one exerts on decisions and recommendations.

Research usually occupies the highest place in hierarchies of evidence. However, simply because something is referred to as research does not give any real indication of its quality. To be an accurate representation of the phenomenon under investigation, research must be carried out using a methodology and methods that are appropriate for the phenomenon being investigated. It must also follow the quality principles for the paradigm which it belongs to and use appropriate methods of data collection and analysis. Poor-quality research or research which uses inappropriate methods of data collection and analysis will not be a useful contribution to the evidence which informs practice.

Expert opinion, case studies, physiological principles, patients' views and cost also contribute to the evidence which informs practice. The place which these occupy in the hierarchy of evidence will depend upon the subject in question, the way in which they have been developed, their quality and the strength of other forms of evidence.

Information that has been gathered from all these sources should be analysed and synthesised so that recommendations can be made regarding the current best evidence on an aspect or aspects of healthcare. These must then be appropriately applied to individual patient situations. Practitioners are required to use their clinical judgement, in conjunction with discussion with patients so as to ascertain their views and preferences, to determine the best course of action in each individual case. The latter two elements of evidence-based practice – using expert clinical judgement and considering the needs and preferences of individuals – are crucial to the provision of quality care, and form an essential part of evidence-based practice. They are not optional extras.

The bear, I am pleased to say, walked free from the scene of the accident.

3

Clinical Guidelines

Clinical guidelines are recommendations, based on the best available evidence, on the appropriate treatment and care for people with specific diseases and conditions (NICE, 2005b). They may be developed with the intention of being used locally or nationally. Although many of the functions of local and national clinical guidelines are similar, there are some distinctions in their remit, their purpose and the issues that they present. This chapter outlines the general purpose, functions and limits of clinical guidelines. Where this is relevant, it discusses how national and local guidelines may differ and the potential problems with, as well as advantages of, using clinical guidelines.

SUMMARIES OF EVIDENCE

Clinical guidelines are intended to be summaries of the current best evidence on aspects of healthcare, presented in a manner that makes the application of evidence to practice clear.

Healthcare professionals are presented with an ever-increasing volume of information on which to base their practice, and it would be difficult, if not impossible, for individuals to gather, appraise and synthesise all the evidence regarding every area of their practice. Staff are often dealing with patients who have multifaceted health related problems that span more than one clinical speciality and include biological, psychological, emotional, social and spiritual needs. At the same time, advances in medicine and technology mean that the range of treatment and interventions available is widening, often rapidly, and creating a population with ever-increasing healthcare requirements. The developments in healthcare span preventative medicine and public health, acute and critical care and long-term or continuing care needs. There is therefore an increasing range of healthcare situations and health conditions about which professionals may be required to find information. It would be unrealistic to expect every practitioner to accomplish the task of knowing everything about every aspect of their practice, even within a clearly delineated speciality. The sheer task of collecting and evaluating all the evidence can be daunting and deter one from even attempting or commencing the task.

Finding information on the kit that I was meant to need for my baby was a challenge, and that was for one newborn baby, whom I assumed would be healthy. Finding evidence on why I was supposed to need each item of equipment which was deemed essential if I was to avoid tragedy, or at least accusations of neglect, was almost impossible. Somewhere, I am sure, there is some evidence on all this. However, I hadn't the time or, really, the inclination to find and read it all. Most of the reports that I saw were from manufacturers. Some advised that your baby was doomed to severe developmental delay or worse unless you invested £100 or more in a plastic product which they had created. If, on the other hand, you invested in their product, your child would be at Oxbridge before he or she was even conceived. Others claimed that children could only really expect to survive the hazardous journey from 0 to 14 if you brought a stash of their inventions and filled your house so full that the child could never move enough to get into danger. He or she would be neatly propped up between boxes of monitoring equipment and safety kit. I bought almost nothing, and my baby has survived so far, but presumably only just.

The range of information on healthcare is hopefully not so biased by manufacturers and emotional blackmail as the 'how to be a halfway decent parent' literature. However, the problem of information overload can still exist. Even in the case of a single patient, the range of treatment and care which is required often means that seeking out, evaluating, synthesising and deciding how to apply the evidence would be hugely time-consuming and the thought of it can be off-putting. For example, for a nurse caring for a child who requires long-term assisted ventilation via a tracheostomy the evidence required would include the optimum mode of ventilation, the best type of tracheostomy tube, the most effective way to provide tracheostomy care and the ideal method of performing suction. These would only involve the respiratory side of the child's care. Additional information would be needed on treatment of the underlying condition which necessitates assisted ventilation. This might include pharmacological management, physiotherapy, surgical interventions and nutrition. Caring for the child and family would also require consideration of the child's development, play, socialisation, facilitation of communication, education and the vast range of the needs of the family. Thus, even in the care of one child, a vast amount of data would need to be collected and evaluated. It would also not be possible or a good use of resources for each member of staff caring for the child to gather, evaluate and synthesise all the information on all these aspects of care.

As well as the sheer range of existing information, how this information is presented can pose a challenge to healthcare staff. Information is available via a wide variety of journals, conferences and electronic media. Electronic availability in some ways increases the convenience with which healthcare staff can access information. It can also make gathering evidence more complex as it means that staff must have the information-retrieval skills needed to gather facts and the skills to evaluate the various forms of evidence presented to them.

Much of the information available to healthcare professionals is also freely available to the public. This ranges from access to full text medical journals to personal websites where individuals offer and share support and advice. Thus, healthcare professionals are likely to be accessing similar or identical resources to those accessed by their patients. Although patients may not have the professional knowledge which professionals have, they may sometimes have superior information-technology and information-retrieval skills. In addition, patients are likely to be accessing a limited subject range of information, for example related to a specific disease or disorder, whereas healthcare staff are often required to access information related to an entire speciality. A member of the public who has a given condition may be very well informed on this, and have accessed all the available information from books, journals, magazines and via the Internet. In contrast, a clinician who may be perceived to be a specialist in the field is likely to have to gather information on this and a range of other diseases, even within their speciality, making their information-gathering remit considerably broader. Nevertheless, there is often an expectation by patients that healthcare professionals will have accessed the full range of information on every subject within their speciality. There is also an increased likelihood that the information provided by healthcare professionals will be challenged by their patients.

The importance of respecting and valuing the knowledge of 'expert patients' is now generally acknowledged (DoH, 2001). However, this can be daunting for staff. Professionals may feel threatened by expert patients, and some parents of children with complex and continuing health needs feel that professionals avoid them for this reason (Glendinning and Kirk, 2000). Shaw and Barker (2004) identify that many medical staff seem to view expert patients as demanding and unreasonable and believe that they tend to present poor-quality information with which to request investigations or treatment.

The relationships between expert patients and healthcare professionals is complex and includes how each party manages the changes in power paradigms and acceptance of different sources and types of knowledge which the idea of patients being experts in their own field brings. Judgements over the perceived quality of information offered by patients must be interpreted in this context. However, one problem with the increased availability of information is that it is not always of high quality, or relevant to all cases even in a broad diagnostic category. For example, Haddow and Watts (2003) found great variability in the quality of information available on the Internet respecting the care required for a febrile child, with much of the information being poor. This is nonetheless the information that is available to the public and on which they may make decisions about the health of their children. There may also be occasions on which patients have access to superior or more up-to-date information than healthcare professionals have. A further challenge can be that the information available, particularly electronically, is international and interventions that are available in other countries or continents may not be available here.

Healthcare professionals therefore need to be able to work with patients, share information and jointly interpret and evaluate this to enable patients to make appropriate informed choices regarding their care. This necessitates staff being familiar with the literature available in their field of practice and its quality, having the communication skills to enable discussions with patients to occur and adopting a mindset in which they are not threatened by their patients accessing information and challenging their views. Chapter 9 discusses in more detail how patient choice is perceived by professionals. However, being aware of the current best evidence is a necessary part of practice and, given the amount of information available, can present a significant challenge to healthcare professionals.

The current enthusiasm for evidence-based practice comes at a time when healthcare professionals have considerable demands on their time, skills and resources. Thus, although the desire to provide care based on the current best evidence may be high, the environment in which professionals must facilitate this is changing and presents multiple and competing priorities. This includes providing direct care, finding information on which to base care, meeting local and national requirements for healthcare provision and audit, and ensuring that documentation and administration are satisfactory.

Given this range of demands and challenges, having available user-friendly summaries of the current best evidence as perceived by experts in the field may assist individual practitioners. It may enable them to base their discussions and practice on the current best evidence within the time constraints that they face. One function of clinical guidelines is therefore to help practitioners in the task of assimilating, evaluating and deciding the clinical application of the vast range of evidence and opinion that is available (SIGN, 2005).

Good-quality guidelines obviate the need for every practitioner to seek out and evaluate the range of information which exists in each speciality. This should enable individuals to practice confidently, knowing that they are providing care which is based on what is thought to be best practice (NHS Modernisation Agency and NICE, 2004a). However, in the same way that not all research is automatically of high quality simply because it is labelled as research, simply labelling something as a guideline gives no guarantee of its quality.

Clinical guidelines are a secondary source of information, as they are a collated summary of the best available evidence, as interpreted by guideline developers. In the majority of cases, practitioners using guidelines will not have read all of the primary sources of evidence or analysed and synthesised these themselves. Chapter 5 discusses how guidelines should be developed and Chapter 6 discusses their evaluation, but it is necessary for practitioners to be aware of the general quality of the clinical guidelines that they use. For example, if a guideline uses out-of-date evidence, limited evidence or poor-quality evidence or is based in how it selects or evaluates evidence, the guidance given will not be good and any care provided based on the guideline will not necessarily be of a high standard. It is therefore useful to have an accepted method of evaluating guideline quality. An international collaboration on clinical guideline development, the AGREE collaboration, has developed an instrument for assessing guideline quality (AGREE, 2001). This represents an accepted standard against which practitioners can evaluate clinical guidelines prior to using them.

PRACTICAL INFORMATION

Clinical guidelines are intended to provide practical guidance for healthcare professionals (Considine and Hood, 2000; Thomas, 1999; SIGN, 2005). They should help to translate theoretical evidence into practice by presenting it in a way that relates to specific clinical situations and that identifies what practitioners should do because of it (Silagy *et al.*, 2001). For example, the RCN guideline on leg ulcers (RCN, 1998) includes information on the methods which should be used to assess, manage, cleanse, débride and dress leg ulcers.

Chapter 1 identified that evidence-based practice is distinct from research in so far as it uses all the current evidence related to a specific element of care. Clinical guidelines take this evidence one step further in that they make statements regarding how the evidence should be applied in specific practice settings or clinical situations. This should mean that practitioners are not presented with abstract theory or principles but have clear and unambiguous statements regarding what care, treatment or intervention should be given, when and how. For example, the RCN guideline on leg ulcer management includes in the assessment section who should perform the assessment, what should be recorded from the history-taking, what should be noted and recorded when examining the patient, what additional observations and investigations should be undertaken, the frequency of reassessment and referral criteria. The evidence which is presented in clinical guidelines or care protocols should also be arranged logically, in a sequence that relates to care provision, so that the guidance given can be followed with comparative ease.

Research usually relates to one aspect of practice, or element of a subject area, and in many cases evidence concerns a similar range of information. Clinical guidelines differ from this in that they may deal with more than one aspect of care. For example, research has been conducted concerning the frequency with which endotracheal suction should be performed, hand hygiene for suctioning, instillation of saline, depth of suction and duration of each suction pass. However, a guideline for performing endotracheal suction would be expected to include all these aspects of performing suction, and to arrange them in a manner which practitioners can easily and logically follow in practice. In some cases, a guideline will deal with the care of an entire condition, for example the NICE guideline on the epilepsies includes investigations, diagnosis, management, review and referral, classification, management of prolonged or repeated seizures in the community, treatment of status epilepticus, people with learning disabilities, young people with epilepsy, older people with epilepsy, people from minority ethnic groups and special considerations for women of childbearing potential (NICE, 2004e). In other cases, a guideline may deal with only one issue within a particular condition, for example the NICE clinical guideline on diabetes: footcare (NICE, 2004f) deals only with this element of diabetic care, although it is complemented by other guidelines on other aspects of diabetic care (NICE, 2002b, 2002c, 2002d, 2002e, 2004g).

The principle of developing a guideline which details the spectrum of care for a given clinical condition, such as the NICE guideline on the management of multiple sclerosis (NICE, 2003e) is congruent with the desire to promote holistic care. However, while including the entire spectrum of patients' needs is a positive step towards the provision of holistic care, this may result in guidelines being unwieldy and off-putting for practitioners. The composite guidance in such documents may be able to be broken down into more easily manageable chunks. For example, the guidance provided for the management of multiple sclerosis is separated into its composite subsections as listed in the guideline, such as diagnosis, treatment, rehabilitation and managing specific impairments. This should enable staff to refer to the relevant part of the document according to what aspect of care they are involved in providing without having to wade through the entire document. The volume of information contained in one document may nonetheless deter busy practitioners from attempting to use it. The balance between providing comprehensive information and providing a volume of information which is unwieldy and off-putting for practitioners is not easy to achieve. Chapter 5 will discuss the need for clear parameters to be decided by guideline developers, but the intention of a clinical guideline is for it to be usable in practice.

For clinical guidelines to be user-friendly, practitioners should also be able to easily identify when they should consider using a guideline. Guidelines should therefore make clear exactly which population they deal with, which procedures, practices, treatment or care they relate to and their limits as well as inclusions. For example, the guidelines issued by NICE on depression in primary and secondary care indicate that they relate to people aged 18 and older with depression being treated in primary and secondary care settings, but that they do not specifically address the diagnosis or treatment of depression in people younger than 18 years or in the context of a separate physical disorder, or dysthymia, seasonal affective disorder or postnatal depression (NICE, 2004d). The NICE guideline on routine care for the healthy pregnant woman indicates that this guidance only pertains to the clinical antenatal care that all healthy women with an uncomplicated singleton pregnancy should receive and baseline care for all pregnancies. It states that it does not cover the additional care that women thought to be at an increased risk of complications should be offered (NICE, 2003d).

SYSTEMATICALLY PREPARED AND PRESENTED INFORMATION

Guidelines should be developed from a systematic evaluation of the current best evidence (NHS Modernisation Agency and NICE, 2004b; Plouffe and Seniuk, 2004; Hughes, 2002; Considine and Hood, 2000). Chapter 5 will discuss the guideline development process, but guidelines should arise from the systematic gathering and evaluation of evidence, and the information in them should be developed and presented systematically (SIGN, 2005). As has been identified previously, the intention is for guidelines to be user-friendly and immediately applicable in practice; they should be presented logically and in a sequence which fits how they will be used. They should also include all aspects of the matter which they are intended to cover so that practitioners who follow them are not left with gaps in care provision. The aim is for them to be presented in a manner that allows practitioners to follow them easily and accurately and to be able to progress logically through care provision.

DECISION-MAKING

Hughes (2002) describes clinical guidelines as tools to aid clinical decision-making. There is some evidence to suggest that decision-making by healthcare professionals does not always match what is deemed to be best practice (Hughes, 2002). If clinical guidelines are of good quality, they therefore have the potential to improve practice by enabling clinicians to make decisions or provide care according to the current best evidence.

As well as enhancing decision-making so that it is in accordance with the current best evidence, clinical guidelines may speed up the decision-making process and enable care to be instituted promptly and to proceed more swiftly and efficiently than would otherwise be the case (Wilcox and Witham, 2003). Whether this is beneficial is dependent on the quality of the clinical guidelines: rapid descisions which are wrong are unlikely to enhance care. However, it is possible that having comprehensive and accessible guidelines will be a useful resource to remind busy staff of the recommended way of dealing with situations, give guidance to staff who are unsure of how to proceeed and allow staff to give treatment or care without potentially dangerous delays.

Good-quality clinical guidelines may also reduce the risk of errors occuring. From data generated between November 2003 and March 2005, errors in the NHS have been identified as accounting for more than 800 deaths per year (Coombes, 2005). Human error is a significant and inevitable aspect of health-care (Morris, 2001). Khan and Hoda (2005) suggest that of the 76% of medical errors that they identified as being preventable, 56% were due to human error rather than systems errors, while the Bristol Inquiry (Kennedy, 2001) suggests that 5% of the 8.5 million people admitted to hospital each year experience a potentially preventable adverse event. Errors are a reality of healthcare. Feied *et al.* (2004) consider that inadequate access to immediate clinical information causes or contributes to many types of medical error. Clinical guidelines may therefore contribute to reducing human error in healthcare by providing staff with a reminder of, or information on, the recommended course of action in a given situation (Wilcox and Witham, 2003). For guidelines to achieve this they must be clear and unambiguous, as their intention to reduce errors will be less likely to be achieved if they are not easy to follow and do not give clear instructions.

In some situations, clinical guidelines include information on which level of staff should manage stages in treatment or care processes. This may be useful as it may contribute to preventing those with insufficient experience or expert-ise from attempting, or feeling coerced to attempt, procedures, processes or activities for which they are insufficiently experienced or skilled. For example, the NICE guideline on the management of multiple sclerosis (NICE, 2003e) states that a consultant neurologist or specialist registrar with suitable expe-rience should discuss the diagnosis of multiple scelerosis with the patient. This has the potential to limit the risk of junior staff either feeling they should or can explore such a diagnosis with patients when they cannot. However, the downside of this is that guidelines may inappropriately limit who is permitted to provide care or carry out elements of care. In a busy service, in which the ideal staffing level and skill mix may not be available, guidelines which strictly prescribe who is and is not permitted to provide treatment or care may mean that care is delayed, which may in turn have an adverse effect on patients. This may be difficult to balance, as unsafe care may be no better than no care, but the pros and cons of recommending which staff should perform which aspects of care must be considered.

Despite their benefits in assisting in decision-making, and reducing errors, as we will discuss in more detail in Chapter 8 clinical guidelines may be con-sidered to impinge upon practitioners' clinical freedom. Dictates over which staff may or may not carry out aspects of care may add to this. Interestingly, this contrasts with the intention of care protocols, which aim to expand, not restrict, the number of staff who are able to provide aspects of care (DoH, 2002). Arguably, the two intentions may be similar, in that care protocols intend to move the focus to the competence of staff to perform procedures rather than focusing on their professional identity. Where guidelines suggest the level of competence, rather than the identity, of the professionals who should carry out care, the two are congruent. However, if the grade or level of staff is indicated, not their ability, these appear to be at odds with one another.

GUIDANCE, NOT RULES

A guideline is defined as 'a general rule, principle, or piece of advice' (Oxford English Dictionary, 2001). Although this definition indicates that a guideline is a rule, it makes clear that it is a **general** rule, not a rigid rule which must be applied in every situation. The intention of clinical guidelines is therefore to provide principles to guide practitioners, not to dictate what must be done (Plouffe and Seniuk, 2004). Clinical guidelines are not intended to be health-care recipies, to be blindly followed regardless of individual circumstances. Rather they aim to provide practitioners with information to assist them in decision-making (SIGN, 2005, NICE, 2005b, Plouffe and Seniuk, 2004). Clinical guidelines provide advice developed by experts in the field based on the evaluation of appropriate evidence. They can include the age, social or cultural group of the patient as well as the disease or condition for which they are designed. However, they cannot identify the specific, diverse and contextual needs of each patient (Witkin and Harrison, 2001). Thus, there is always a need to consider how appropriate any guidance is in individual cases. This includes considering coexisting pathology, the variety of diagnostic and interventional procedures being performed, individual patient preferences and their social circumstances, beliefs and life priorities.

To return to my feckless hiking in dangerous situations, we usually carry reasonable medical kit with us on big hikes when we are days from what passes for civilisation. This includes bits and pieces of medication to stop the injured from whingeing and spoiling the views. I am not sure what the actual recommendation for non-steroidal anti-inflammatory drugs in this situation is. Possibly that we should be sympathetic rather than medicate, and possibly ibuprofen if sympathy fails and drugs are needed clinically rather than socially. We carry Voltarol, mainly because we are not really very sympathetic, secondly because it is smaller and lighter than ibuprofen and, finally, if you get it wet it creates heroic muddy stains on your pack, suggestive of adventure and engagement with mud, not pink girly smears suggestive of carrying lippy on the trail. Our priorities are kind of medical in the outcome of analgesia and anti-inflammatory properties, and Voltarol is a pretty effective drug for that I guess, but size, weight and general image are the key things. This is possibly not the way in which a physician or pharmacist would view the evidence and make decisions about prescribing, and any of those folk reading this may be having a nasty moment just now, but it does very nicely for me.

There are also likely to be cases where a patient requires care which involves more than one guideline. For instance, a guideline may be used for weaning patients from mechanical ventilation. However, patients being weaned from assisted ventilation may also require pain control and endotracheal suctioning. In some cases, the steps advocated in these guidelines may be incongruent with one another and healthcare staff will be required to prioritise and determine which aspect of each guideline is the most important at any given time and how the steps advocated in each guideline complement or contradict one another.

Good-quality clinical guidelines may be a useful resource to assist in providing high standards of care, and be an aid to decision-making, but they cannot, of themselves, guarantee quality care or good decision-making. To achieve this, they must be used in conjunction with consideration of an individual patient's needs and circumstances.

ASSIST IN THE PROVISION OF QUALITY CARE

One of the intentions of clinical guidelines is to improve the quality of care provided by enabling staff to base their practice on the current best evidence. However, having a clinical guideline in existence does not provide any guarantee that the quality of care will be improved.

First of all, a guideline must be of good quality to produce good care. It must also be accessible to practitioners and be used in appropriate circumstances. Chapter 7 discusses the processes by which guideline implementation may be improved, and Chapters 8 and 9 discuss how clinical expertise and patient choice can be incorporated into guideline use. These are all necessary considerations if clinical guidelines are to enhance practice.

Although it is clearly stated by individuals and national guideline development groups such as NICE and SIGN that guidelines should inform, not dictate, practice, there may be a conflict of purpose in this respect as one of the aims of the development of national guidelines is to increase the equity of healthcare across geographical regions (NICE, 2004i). This will be discussed further in later chapters, but it is a potential contradiction in national clinical guidelines.

STANDARDISATION OF PRACTICE

The Bristol Inquiry (Kennedy, 2001) recommended that clear national guidance and standards of practice should be developed. Further to this, the DoH (2000) have also stated their intention to improve the equity of healthcare provision. The development of national clinical guidelines, such as those developed by NICE, may assist in achieving this objective. Although NICE state that their guidance is intended to inform, not dictate, practice, a part of the reason for NICE being required to develop national clinical guidelines is to promote consistency of care across geographical regions. This may enhance equity of access to healthcare, based on the current best evidence, and ensure that all individuals have access to equal standards, and methods, of healthcare provision, regardless of their location (NICE, 2004i). It may also be considered to be a fairer approach to healthcare provision, especially in light of the many demands which exist for a publicly funded national health service. Having clinical guidelines available may make clear to the public what they can expect and what the limits, as well as inclusions, on provision are. However, they may also mean that some choices are not available, or are available only with difficulty, for some patients and that clinicians do not in fact have the freedom to offer some treatment or care options which they might wish to. Their remit in relation to a national standardisation of care may also introduce a degree of duress for practitioners to conform to them. Chapters 8, 9, 10 and 11 will discuss the issues related to professional autonomy, client choice, cost and the political elements of clinical guidelines and care protocols in more detail. However, despite NICE's overriding statement on every guideline it issues that clinical guidelines must be used in conjunction with individual expertise and patient choice, this may be problematic. There may be a conflict of purpose where clinical guidelines are related to quality-assurance statements and where adherence to them is taken as a measure of achieving quality care. Thus, while on the one hand clinical guidelines may be used as indicators of good practice, they may also limit practitioners' freedom to provide what they and their patients perceive to be high-quality care for individuals.

MEASURING PRACTICE

Clinical guidelines have a role in achieving quality in care provision by giving guidance on what is deemed to be the best approach to care. They can also fulfil a role in the evaluation and auditing of care. As clinical guidelines should clearly outline the recommended steps to be taken at each stage in a given situation, they should also be able to be used as a tool to measure whether or not these steps have been followed. This applies to both local and national guidelines (NHS Modernisation Agency and NICE, 2004a). Although this may seem to be a logical method of assessing the quality of care provision, it increases the potential for clinical guidelines to be seen as rules which must be followed, or which must be followed if individuals or organisations are to be deemed to have achieved best practice. It also assumes that following a clinical guideline is equal to the provision of good-quality care.

Monitoring quality is an important part of healthcare (DoH, 1998), and auditing standards of practice in order to protect the public is considered to be essential (Kennedy, 2001). However, while auditing the implementation of clinical guidelines is important, the actual quality of care, not simply whether the guidelines are used, is what is important (Hewitt-Taylor, 2003). Chapters 5 and 6 look in more detail at how guidelines should be used and evaluated, but there is a risk that evaluation will only be of whether a guideline was used, not its quality, the reasons for any failure to implement it or outcomes of care as a result of guideline use or non-use. It may be that a clinical guideline is impractical or of poor quality. In such instances, adhering to it would be inappropriate or even unsafe. Rather than simply recording whether or not the guideline was used, the rationale for non-use where this is the case should be ascertained so that the practicality of the guidance and the actual quality issue can be assessed rather than simply the guideline's usage.

EDUCATION

It has been suggested that clinical guidelines can be used as an education and training tool for healthcare professionals (NHS Modernisation Agency and NICE, 2004a). They can be used to instruct students or for post-registration education and in-service training. By providing an outline of the current best evidence they may be useful in teaching about procedures, care situations, diseases or disorders. However, the extent to which they will be useful in facilitating high-quality education depends upon how they are used. If they are used as a tool to state what must be done and why, they may serve a useful purpose in enabling healthcare professionals to understand what is recommended and the reason for this. However, while this kind of procedural teaching may be useful in some instances, for example where the aim is simply to instruct individuals on a given procedure, it is more akin to training than education, and to rote learning, not inquiry. This will not particularly contribute to a questioning approach to practice or the development of critically aware practitioners who can apply guidance appropriately to individual situations.

There have been suggestions that focusing on clinical guidelines may detract from healthcare staff developing expertise or decision-making skills if they become used to their decision trail being dictated or presented to them. Clinical guidelines can nonetheless be useful for education, particularly if this includes looking beyond the prescribed guidance. Education can involve discussion of how evidence was sought, evaluated and synthesised and the critical exploration of the process of guideline development and any resultant guidance. Education can also include debate about the quality and content of specific guidelines, the potential conflicts in their use, the way in which individual needs and choices can be incorporated into guideline use, and political and resource issues. This may contribute to the development of a workforce that is able to critically analyse their own practice and adopt an analytical approach to decision-making. However, whether clinical guidelines and care protocols are useful in the development of critically aware practitioners who are aware of real world conflicts, or detract from practitioners developing decision-making skills, depends, to a great extent, on how they are used.

COMMUNICATION WITH PATIENTS

The NHS Modernisation Agency and NICE (2004a) and SIGN (2005) suggest that clinical guidelines may be a useful tool for facilitating communication between healthcare staff and patients. Having clinical guidelines available may help patients to know what they can expect from the healthcare system, and what the consensus is on what constitutes best practice. This is congruent with the recommendations made by the Bristol Inquiry (Kennedy, 2001). It has also been suggested that clinical guidelines can help patients to make informed decisions about their treatment or care as they will be aware of the available options, and why these are recommended (SIGN, 2005; NHS Modernisation Agency and NICE, 2004a). This may be especially helpful where conflicting advice exists, where patients have accessed information which is out of date or inaccurate, or where treatment has not been recommended as a good use of NHS resources, despite some patients wanting it. While it could be argued that clinical guidelines decrease patient choices by limiting the available options, they may make clearer what the existing options are and why this is and deflect responsibility for apparently withholding treatment from individual practitioners. It may also be helpful for patients who feel that the care or treatment they have received is not appropriate to be able to see whether this is supported by clinical guidelines on the subject. For example, the NICE clinical guidelines on Caesarean section may reassure women who have been advised against a Caesarean section on request that this is in line with recommended best practice, and thought to be in their best interests and the best interests of their babies (NICE, 2004h).

The NHS Modernisation Agency and NICE (2004a) suggest that clinical guidelines can thus improve communication between patients and healthcare professionals by providing a fixed frame of reference from which discussions can proceed. This may well be the case, but it is largely dependent upon whether guidelines are viewed as guidance, open to debate between professional and patient, or rigid rules, which must be followed and of which patients are informed, and not from which joint discussion emerges. It also depends on the communication skills of the professionals involved. Guidelines cannot, of themselves, alter the interpersonal skills of individuals. If individual healthcare professionals are impolite, disrespectful of patients' needs or views or fail to listen to patients, clinical guidelines cannot alter their basic behaviour. A nurse may use a clinical guideline as a tool to guide sensitive discussion and informed decision-making regarding care. Equally, they may use a clinical guideline to brusquely inform a patient of what will happen. Similarly, if patients are unwilling to listen to the opinions of professionals, or are aggressive or impolite, clinical guidelines being available to facilitate discussion will not necessarily alter an individual's approach to communication.

SUMMARY

Clinical guidelines should be user-friendly summaries of the current best evidence related to aspects of healthcare. They should be systematically developed and presented so as to provide clear guidance on the steps to be taken in given situations. They may aid decision-making by outlining what is the recommended course of action in certain circumstances. However, the advice which they give must be interpreted in conjunction with an assessment of each patient's individual needs.

The intention of clinical guidelines is to guide, rather than direct, practice. However, because they offer a mechanism by which adherence to the recommended processes and procedures can be monitored, this may be problematic. Measuring the use of clinical guidelines will only determine whether or not the steps which they recommend have been followed, not the actual quality of care. Monitoring the use of clinical guidelines may contribute to auditing care and will be useful if used in conjunction with other measures of care provision. However, apparent guideline use does not, of itself, give a reliable indication of the quality of care and does not necessarily reflect whether or not patients believe that they have received a high standard of care. Many complaints about healthcare concern aspects of communication, which cannot be precisely described in guideline statements, for example tone of voice, respect and listening skills. Clinical guidelines may be a useful communication tool for patients to be made aware of what they can expect from healthcare providers, their choices, and the limits of their choices, and to provide a frame of reference for discussion. They may provide a useful aid to communication between healthcare professionals and patients, but they cannot replace good communication skills.

Clinical guidelines may be a useful adjunct to the education and training of healthcare professionals, and may be a valuable tool around which to structure teaching about certain conditions or interventions. However, their value in terms of education rather than training and the development of critically aware expert practitioners will depend upon the manner in which they are used.

4

Care Protocols

Care protocols are detailed descriptions of the steps which should be taken to deliver treatment or care (NHS Modernisation Agency and NICE, 2004a). They should provide practitioners with evidence-based information which clearly states what should be done, when, how and by whom. Care protocols may relate to diseases, for example protocols dealing with diabetes or asthma, problems, for example chest pain and anxiety, be based on treatments, for example hip replacement, or be based on client groups, for example people with learning disabilities or neonates (NHS Modernisation Agency, 2004a). Comparing this definition with the definition of clinical guidelines provides very little indication of a difference between the two, and there is often a lack of clarity over the distinction between care protocols, clinical guidelines and care pathways. In many cases, the terms are used interchangeably, and this may not be important, as many of the issues involved are very similar. However, it is worth noting the distinctions which exist between these terms.

This chapter therefore defines care protocols and discusses the differences between these, clinical guidelines and care pathways. It then discusses the purposes, advantages and challenges presented by care protocols. Because of the similarities between clinical guidelines and care protocols, the points made regarding care protocols are often the same as, or very similar to, those for clinical guidelines. In these cases, the discussion is not repeated, and the debate in Chapter 3 is referred to.

CARE PROTOCOLS AND CLINICAL GUIDELINES

Like clinical guidelines, care protocols may be developed locally or nationally. Their intention, like that of clinical guidelines, is to provide evidence-based information in a format which makes it immediately usable in practice settings. However, care protocol documents tend to be less extensive than clinical guidelines and detail the steps to be taken more succinctly and with less detail of rationale. Care protocols should be derived from a similar trawling of the current best evidence as clinical guidelines, and should be informed by a significant volume of information, but less information is usually included in the protocol document itself. They are often confined to one or two A4 sheets, so that they can be conveniently displayed and referred to easily in practice situations. In some cases, clinical guidelines include summaries within them, for example the NICE guideline on preoperative testing (NICE, 2003f) includes a summary in A4 format. However, clinical guideline documents are usually presented in greater depth and have more supporting information contained in them. Care protocols may be included in clinical guideline documents, for example a clinical guideline on management of aggression in accident and emergency departments might include a protocol for the restraint of patients.

Although the NHS Modernisation Agency and NICE (2004a) state that protocols may be disease based, problem based, client based or treatment based, they tend to be developed for specific elements of care. This is not an absolute distinction, but the tendency is for protocols to be developed in areas that are amenable to procedures being reduced to a staged description. It would be difficult to develop a protocol for care of a neonate, but a bank of protocols related to neonatal care might be developed, for example a protocol for caring for an infant who requires phototherapy, a protocol for administering fluids to a neonate, a protocol for sedation of a critically ill neonate. One of the potential problems with such a bank of protocols is that this may result in care being seen as reducible to following a series of protocols, with scant attention given to the care which links the protocols and addresses individual needs. Chapters 8 and 9 will discuss this issue in more detail. However, the content of clinical guidelines being more extensive and detailed than care protocols increases the likelihood of them being able to convey the importance of holistic care.

Nationally, care protocols are similar to clinical guidelines in so far as NICE produce national clinical guidelines and the NHS Modernisation Agency and NICE (2004b) suggest that care protocols should be based around their guidance or other recognised standards. Their development is a requirement in relation to achieving the standards set out in some National Service Frameworks (NHS Modernisation Agency and NICE, 2004b) and the DoH (2000) have stated that healthcare staff in England should be using nationally agreed care protocols which dictate the recommended treatment or care for common clinical conditions. Care protocols are therefore also a part of a national agenda that is linked with the achievement of quality standards. However, unlike clinical guidelines, there is no national centre for protocol development akin to NICE and SIGN. The NHS Modernisation Agency and NICE (2004b) provide information on protocols and how these may be developed but do not have a bank of care protocols or a system for their development as they do with clinical guidelines. The NHS Modernisation Agency has a team which aims to help identify and implement ways of realising the Government's commitment to develop and spread the use of protocol-based care and the National Electronic Library for Health has a 'Protocols and Care Pathways' database and provides a national point of access for sharing and disseminating care protocols and integrated care pathways. However, protocols from the National Electronic Library for Health do not currently hold the same status as NICE guidelines and the organisation does not have the authority which NICE does for issuing guidance to the NHS.

CARE PROTOCOLS AND CARE PATHWAYS

The NHS Modernisation Agency and NICE (2004a) state that care protocols are often also described as care pathways, or integrated care pathways. However, there are distinctions between these two types of document (National Electronic Library for Health, 2005). The National Electronic Library for Health (2005) indicates that care pathways may include clinical guidelines or care protocols but that each are distinct entities. They suggest that, unlike clinical guidelines or care protocols, care pathways record deviations from planned care or recommended procedures as well as giving a prescription for them. They describe care pathways as being like care protocols or clinical guidelines in so far as they aim to identify who should do what, when and in what order. However, unlike care protocols or clinical guidelines, care pathways include a record of the outcome in each particular instance of use, or the patient's individual experience. Care protocols and clinical guidelines should be evaluated (NHS Modernisation Agency and NICE, 2004b), and only used where they are appropriate for individual patient's needs. However, care pathways relate to individual patients, tend to deal with their entire experience and include a comparison of planned care with care actually given in specific cases. Thus, although the terms 'care protocol' and 'care pathway' may be used interchangeably in some texts, and have a great deal in common, they are not synonymous (National Electronic Library for Health, 2005).

For instance, a care pathway for the care of a patient with cancer might include a care protocol on the recommended procedure for the administration of chemotherapy. However, it would also include a place to record whether this was administered as planned, the extent of the side effects, the patient's response and any additional observations. It would also include sections on other aspects of care, such as any reference to or inclusion of a clinical guideline on pain management and/or a care protocol on any emetic administration. The care pathway would therefore represent a holistic picture of the patient's pathway of treatment and care, as prescribed but also as delivered and experienced by that patient.

GUIDANCE OR RULES?

One of the major differences between care protocols and clinical guidelines is the degree of obligation that they carry. Care protocols, like clinical guidelines, aim to provide practitioners with evidence-based information which clearly demonstrates the best method of care provision in specific situations (Considine and Hood, 2000). However, unlike guidelines, protocols are described as 'the official procedure or system of rules . . . the accepted code of behaviour in a particular situation' (Oxford English Dictionary, 2001). These may therefore be interpreted as fixed steps or procedures that must be followed in all cases. This contrasts a little with clinical guidelines which are consistently described as general rules, not absolute rules (NICE, 2005b; SIGN, 2005). Care protocols are therefore more likely to be seen as non-negotiable requirements, and assumed to be, from their name, prescriptive of what must be done.

Protocols can result in inflexible behaviour, dependent on the practitioner using them, as we found out on a trip across North America. It is not permitted to take fruit from Canada to the USA or vice versa, but we had somehow remained in ignorance of this until we reached a small border crossing in North Dakota. We were carrying forbidden bananas for our lunch (which we would be stopping for just the other side of the border checkpoint, within view of the customs house). The Canadian customs officer smiled at us and our weary-looking fruit stash (which had travelled the 24 hours from Chicago on a Greyhound bus) and allowed us to lunch in peace, possibly because he felt that anyone who was inclined to carry a banana that far on a Greyhound bus was dangerously insane and best left alone. Our luck and fruit's fate were very different when we entered Seattle from Victoria. After our ferry crossing, we were headed towards a twelve-hour Greyhound bus ride, to Santa Cruz, and had a small stash of luncheon with us to stave off McDonald's and hunger. A large customs official bore down on us and asked if we were importing any fruit. We had, for some reason, not remembered that fruit imports were banned and confessed to having an apple and a pear. The official drew himself up to his full height and puffed himself out to his full breadth and looked at us as if we were a mutated life form somehow combined of Osama Bin Laden and an amoeba. 'Importing fruit is forbidden by federal law,' he informed us, handling his gun as he spoke. 'You are in contravention of federal law for attempting to bring this into the USA.' We handed over our fruit. It didn't seem worth dying for. The defender of Federal Law marched off, holding the sadly crumpled paper bag of illegal imports away from him, presumably to avoid contamination. His expression implied a bad smell under his nose and his moustache bristled with indignation. I am not sure if we will be allowed back into the USA later this year, as we may be included on the database of individuals who have done the kind of thing that means that George Bush is not keen on them. The point, in relation to protocols, is that the Canadian and American had the same protocol, and of course the American was right. But in neither case did fruit really cross the border, in any meaningful sense, and I know whose 'care' I was more satisfied with.

The suggestion that protocols are more akin to rules which must be followed means that they have a greater potential to decrease a practitioner's perceived ability to use their clinical judgement and take into account individual circumstances or needs. However, as Chapter 8 will identify, medico-legally, neither care protocols nor clinical guidelines remove or reduce a practitioner's responsibility to use their clinical judgement or to address individual client need when providing care.

Although care protocols may be perceived as detrimental to professional autonomy, that they imply a degree of obligation need not be a negative point. It may be that by developing agreed protocols staff are enabled or permitted to provide care which they might otherwise not feel confident to provide or might feel could not be justified as a use of resources, despite its potential benefits. For example, Buss *et al.* (2004) describe a situation in which the Southampton Memory Services Commissioners were concerned about the cost-effectiveness of using cholinesterase inhibitors, despite NICE recommending their use. A formal prescribing protocol was therefore developed, with one reason for its development being that it was felt that it would help to reassure the commissioners that the local service would act responsibly and within set parameters in prescribing these drugs. Thus, having a protocol enabled care provision to proceed, with practitioners having the authority to prescribe drugs which they might otherwise have been inhibited from using.

EVIDENCE-BASED INFORMATION

Like clinical guidelines, care protocols are intended to provide practitioners with easily accessible evidence-based guidance, thus improving the information available to them (NHS Modernisation Agency and NICE, 2004a). This comes with similar caveats to those identified in Chapter 3 in that the information provided in protocols will only be as good as the information on which the protocol is predicated and the process by which it was developed. A document being described as a care protocol does not guarantee that it is of high quality or that using it will produce safe or high-quality care.

Practitioners should evaluate care protocols to determine their quality prior to using them, in the same way that they should with clinical guidelines. The NHS Modernisation Agency and NICE (2004b) have issued guidance on the development of care protocols, and the AGREE (2001) standards which can be used to assess the quality of clinical guidelines outlined in Chapter 5 can, to an extent, also be applied to care protocols. However, because care protocol documents tend to be shorter than clinical guidelines, with less detail of how and by whom they were developed, the types of evidence used and the hierarchies into which these were placed, evaluating them may be less easy to achieve. In most cases, the intention of protocols is that they are succinct documents which can be followed rapidly and step-by-step in practice, in a manner akin to a quick reference guide. Thus, their comparatively reduced volume of information is appropriate to their purpose. However, although the document which is presented as a care protocol is likely to be brief, information regarding the way in which evidence was gathered, evaluated and synthesised to develop the protocol should be available. This may mean the protocol providing direction to a fuller document on the development process. How guidelines and protocols can best be introduced into practice will be discussed in Chapter 11, but their introduction should include the involvement of the staff who will be using them. Explanations of why, how and by whom they have been developed should be included in the discussions, education and training specific to implementing any care protocol.

The existence of a care protocol or clinical guideline does not remove a practitioner's responsibility for making appropriate decisions about specific care situations. Information on the quality of any care protocol which it is suggested that practitioners use therefore needs to be available in some format so that staff can make, and assist patients to make, informed decisions.

As discussed previously, care protocols tend to be more brief and directive than clinical guidelines. Consequently, despite being more prescriptive, they may be more useful in acute situations where a busy practitioner is confronted with clinical need and wishes to know, swiftly, what is thought to be the best thing to do and how to do this. By providing easily usable, staged, instructions, care protocols may contribute to the reduction of errors and increase the efficacy and safety of care (NHS Modernisation Agency and NICE, 2004a; Morris, 2001; Wall *et al.*, 2001). Like clinical guidelines, care protocols are likely to be especially useful in situations where all staff members may not be aware of the composite current best evidence (Campbell *et al.*, 1998) and for staff who are relatively inexperienced in a particular field of practice or aspect of care. For example, in an accident and emergency department, it may be useful for staff who are not experienced in dealing with children to have a protocol for treating croup which gives clear, step-by-step information on what to include in assessing the child, acceptable and unacceptable physiological parameters, drug doses, when to refer a child and to whom. Chapter 8 deals in more detail with the professional and legal aspects of clinical guideline and care protocol use, but there are situations where there is little time for debate on what should be done, or where specialist intervention is being awaited but a patient must be stabilised in the interim period. There are also situations where patients will be cared for in a ward or department outside the speciality to which they 'belong'. This may be because an individual has a disease with multisystem involvement or because they are awaiting transfer or bed availability. For instance, the recommendation is that children who require intensive care should usually be cared for in a designated PICU (DoH, 1997). However, even where a child is of a dependancy level that requires definite admission to a

PICU, unless they become ill in or near a lead centre, they will need to be stabilised and await transfer to a regional PICU. Given the geographical spread of PICUs, this may take some time. In such situations, approved protocols may allow practitioners who must care for the child to proceed with care provision in relative safety until retrieval to a regional centre can be effected.

IMPROVED CARE

The NHS Modernisation Agency and NICE (2004a) claim that, by providing accessible, evidence-based information, care protocols can promote high-quality, effective care. There is some evidence that the use of protocols related to specific interventions can improve clinical outcomes (Morris *et al.*, 2001). For example, Brook *et al.* (1999) report that the use of a protocol for sedation reduced the length of time that patients spent in intensive care. McKendry *et al.* (2004) describe how a protocol for optimising circulatory status in patients who had undergone cardiac surgery reduced complications and shortened their stay in both intensive care and hospital. Dries *et al.* (2004) suggest that a protocol for weaning from mechanical ventilation reduced the use of assisted ventilation and the number of failed extubations. Using care protocols therefore has the potential to enhance care and patient outcomes. As stated previously, this tends to mean that the use of care protocols improves care in relation to specific procedures or means that isolated aspects of care become more effective or efficient. For a patient's overall care to be improved, the individual aspects of care which are covered by protocols must be embedded in a care experience which seeks to meet each individual's multifaceted needs.

The DoH (2000) also intend that national care protocols will enable a wider range of staff to provide certain aspects of care. The suggestion is that, by outlining what should be done and what interventions or procedures are required in a given situation, any person who is competent to carry these out can provide care, regardless of their professional identity. This may be beneficial in reducing the number of staff with whom patients come into contact and in some instances may mean that one member of staff can provide all the necessary care. This should, logically, lead to more individualised and holistic care as the care provider will be able to get to know the patient, discuss their treatment and care with them and organise for this to happen in a timeframe and sequence which is best for the individual. It may also speed up care by reducing the time spent in liaison between staff and waiting for a range of professionals to see a patient. In this way, care protocols may reduce cost, reduce length of hospitalisation and improve the quality of the care experience for the patient. A nurse being able to admit a patient, order investigations, carry out certain investigative procedures and treatments and prescribe drugs within certain parameters may mean that these elements of care can be carried out more promptly than if a range of professionals needed to be involved. In intensive care, a protocol for weaning from mechanical ventilation may allow patients to be weaned more rapidly, without recourse to unnecessary medical review and the delays which this might cause, and thus reduce the duration of intubation and assisted ventilation and the risks associated with this. However, protocol use can give rise to concerns over the reduction of care to a series of tasks or procedures in which the 'whole person' is lost and the assumption that all that is needed to perform care is the technical skills to carry out procedures.

The NHS Modernisation Agency and NICE (2004a) also claim that the use of protocols enhances the continuity and consistency of care and streamlines care provision by reducing unnecessary duplication, particularly between different departments and different care providers. Their use also should ensure that the treatment or care which a patient is receiving is not changed frequently, possibly before an intervention has the chance to become effective. It should also enable staff to easily hand over what stage of a care protocol has been reached when a patient is transferred to another department or when another individual or team takes over their care. This should contribute towards avoiding confusion and unnecessary delays or replication of interventions. Achieving this kind of consistency nonetheless requires all organisations or departments involved in an individual's care to be using the same protocol. For example, a protocol for the care of an infant with meningococcal disease may be developed by a paediatric intensive care team in a lead centre. However, given that a large number of referrals will be from outside the hospital in which the PICU is located and may even be from outside the region, how far the care protocol promotes consistency of care depends upon how widely it is circulated and agreed to. It is likely that it will promote consistency of care within the unit, but infants and children may have different treatment initiated prior to admission and some degree of regional or national standardisation of care protocols may therefore be very desirable.

STANDARDISATION OF CARE

Like clinical guidelines, care protocols are intended to provide some degree of standardisation of care and, if developed nationally, to contribute to equal national standards of care (Considine and Hood, 2000; DoH, 2000; NHS Modernisation Agency and NICE, 2004a). The development of national care protocols is therefore in line with the government's aims to improve the equality of care provision across the country (DoH, 1998). To this end, the DoH's (2000) intention is that national care protocols will be developed and used so that all staff, regardless of their professional identity or location, will follow the same protocol. The intention of this move is that the same standard of care will be provided to all individuals, regardless of who is providing it or where it is provided. One problem with this approach is that it assumes that equity of care can be achieved by following set processes or procedures. A theme which runs through this book is that there is much more to care provision than following procedures. While all staff working in broad accordance with set protocols may give some degree of equity of care provision, there are a vast range of vital aspects of care which affect quality, which cannot be reduced to the stages outlined in care protocols. Joe Simpson, the climber made famous by walking for four days to base camp with a broken leg, after he was assumed to have died, said, 'There is no protocol for telling your friend that you are leaving him to die.' (Moore, 2005). Similarly, there can be no protocol or absolute clinical guideline for telling a parent that their child has a profound disability, for telling a fit young man that he has a progressive disorder which means he will become dependent on others or for telling a patient with cancer that all the treatment options have been tried, without success. There may be guidance on certain aspects of this, such as the importance of an unhurried environment, privacy, the opportunity to have family members present during discussions and observing the verbal and non-verbal cues of the patient. However, the personal and individual nature of this experience and responses to it means that it cannot be reduced to a neatly stated protocol. There can also be no protocol for how a patient should be touched by medical and nursing staff, how they are spoken to and how their dignity and humanity are respected. Thus, the actual standard or quality of care provision between patients cannot be made equal by the use of protocols. The use of a care protocol may mean that the same medical and technical procedures or treatment are offered to all patients, but cannot, of itself, provide total equality in the standard or quality of care provision.

DECISION-MAKING

By outlining the course of action which should be taken, care protocols are intended to assist healthcare staff in decision-making. However, like clinical guidelines, how the use of care protocols will affect staff's decision-making abilities is not clear. Considine and Hood (2000) identify that care protocols are intended to guide and facilitate, not replace, clinical decision-making. However, there is a fear that overuse of care protocols will impair the development and maintenance of clinical judgement (Wall *et al.*, 2001). The evolution of a healthcare culture in which it is expected that the majority of aspects of care can be delivered in accordance with a pre-specified protocol is not an attractive idea. This would be detrimental to staff developing or retaining the ability to assess and evaluate individual need or to provide care which falls outside the boundaries of existing guidelines or protocols. There is a risk that the perception may develop that the only decision needed is which care protocol to use rather than identifying and framing decisions in accordance with individual circumstances and variations in the precise clinical condition of patients. There is a risk that this will produce a generation of care providers who cannot weigh up alternatives and make their own decisions. It does not mean that the best method of providing a single aspect of care should not be identified and recommended for use, for example certain technical and pharmacological aspects of care such as setting up total parenteral nutrition or performing suction may be usefully guided by protocols. However, there is a distinction between using care protocols in conjunction with professional expertise to make decisions in each case as to the precise best course of action and protocol-driven care in which a rigid set of procedures are followed without consideration of the multiple factors impinging on what would be best practice in each specific case.

QUALITY ASSURANCE

The NHS Modernisation Agency and NICE (2004a) state that using care protocols contributes to the achievement of high standards of care by providing a standard against which practice can be measured. This is a similar situation to the use of clinical guidelines in relation to quality assurance. Whether protocols are available and are used can indeed be monitored as a form of quality measurement. A number of NHS organisations are already required to produce protocols as part of the implementation of National Service Frameworks, for example all secondary-care providers should have had protocols for the management of coronary heart disease in place since April 2001, ambulance services should have had protocols for the management of acute myocardial infarction since April 2001 and primary care should have had protocols for the secondary prevention of coronary heart disease, heart failure and rehabilitation since April 2002 (NHS Modernisation Agency and NICE, 2004a). Thus, checking whether care protocols are used can be a tool to measure whether what is deemed to be an adequate standard of care is being provided, and their development or existence may be considered to demonstrate whether an organisation is making adequate progress towards central targets for healthcare provision. Nonetheless, as with clinical guidelines, the existence of care protocols and their use will, of itself, only show whether a care protocol exists or was used, not the outcomes of care, the quality of care provided or patient satisfaction with care. It will also only provide information on one aspect of care. For example, an NHS Trust may have developed and implemented impressive protocols for the secondary prevention of coronary heart disease. However, they may have spent a great deal of time and resources on this, which may mean that their provision for elderly care has suffered. While care may be visibly and measurably improved in one area, this provides no indication or guarantee that care across the board is enhanced. It also only indicates if protocols are used, not if they are used appropriately.

MULTIDISCIPLINARY WORKING

The DoH (2000) and the NHS Modernisation Agency and NICE (2004a) suggest that using protocol-based care gives staff greater opportunities to work in ways to make the best use of their skills, knowledge and expertise and provides a framework for working in multidisciplinary teams. As was identified earlier in this chapter, it has been suggested that by specifying the skills and knowledge needed to carry out specific roles, rather than the care activities which individuals are allowed to carry out depending on their professional identity, care protocols have the potential to increase individuals' scope of practice. This may enable some staff, such as nurses, to carry out a wider range of activities and thus achieve greater autonomy in caseload management than has previously been possible (DoH, 2002). This also accords with the DoH's (2000) aim for healthcare professionals to be trained to work more flexibly, across traditional professional and organisational boundaries. Care protocols are intended to play a part in this increase in role flexibility as they will provide information relevant to specific situations which can be used by a number of disciplines. The suggestion is that, as well as this role expansion enhancing care by exposing patients to fewer healthcare staff, it will improve job satisfaction for many healthcare professionals by increasing their autonomy as they will, in some cases, be able to provide an entire care programme for individual patients, without recourse to other professions. However, Jones and Davies (1999) have identified the possibility that nurses' role expansion will be reduced to taking on additional skills or tasks from other professions which do little to develop the nursing care which patients receive. This is discussed in more detail in Chapter 11; however, although implementing care protocols may enable a greater range of staff to carry out specific procedures, how far providing care in accordance with a series of protocols enhances professional autonomy and job satisfaction is debatable.

COMMUNICATION

The NHS Modernisation Agency and NICE (2004a) claim that using care protocols improves the quality, speed and effectiveness with which information is given to patients, and that this supports their involvement in decision-making and enhances the quality of consent. In many respects, the issues related to communication are the same with care protocols as those, discussed in Chapter 3, regarding clinical guidelines. However, as care protocols are more procedure-related than guidelines, it is more likely that they will be used to assist practitioners to outline to patients the procedures which will be followed if they consent to treatment, or the various options available and how these will be carried out. This means that they may enable patients to understand what will happen, when and how rather than the complexities of the relative risks of various treatment options, the risk versus benefit of interventions and why treatment or care options are or are not recommended.

To return to our fruit crimes, the rules on fruit movement also apply to many Australian states. However, you are usually advised of any forthcoming fruit removal points and why this is (to prevent the spread of fruit flies). Pretty generally, on Australian Greyhound buses, you are also woken half an hour before the fruit confiscation point and reminded to eat any outstanding fruit. The fruit-confiscating American, the lunch-permitting Canadian and the protocol-explaining Australians all have protocols to follow, all of which are more or less the same, and in no case is fruit really allowed across the border. But the methods of communication we experienced were very different every time.

Care protocols, like clinical guidelines, may be a useful starting point for discussions and a helpful guide or prompt sheet to ensure that nothing is forgotten. However, in the same way that following a protocol provides no guarantee of quality of care, they provide no guarantee of quality of discussion or consent. Indeed, the aim of improving informed consent may itself be somewhat counterproductive, as the aim is for patients to make informed decisions, not necessarily to consent to any given intervention or to the steps outlined in a protocol. Consent implies agreeing to treatment, interventions or procedures. Informed choice, in which consent is given or withheld, is perhaps a more appropriate aim.

RESEARCH

Morris (2001) suggests that using care protocols enables rigorous clinical research to be undertaken. Where protocols are used in everyday practice it can be assumed with reasonable confidence that the treatment or care which is routinely given is the same regardless of which practitioner is providing it. This means that if research is being undertaken on a group of patients in which an experimental group and control group exists, aspects of care that are covered by protocols should be the same, meaning that the confidence with which any differences in outcome can be attributed to the experimental intervention is increased. For example, if a new drug, which is being researched, is being used as a chemoprophylaxis for gastric ulceration in patients in intensive care, provided the same feeding protocol is being used for all patients, it could be assumed with reasonable confidence that the feeding which patients received does not affect study outcomes.

Although this may be the case, all positivist research should take into account variables which might exist, and most positivist research should itself include protocols which attempt to reduce the variables between subjects. If research is being conducted, it will still be necessary to ascertain that all staff are adhering to any requisite care protocols and that any existing care protocols fit the intentions of the research, rather than assuming this to be the case.

SUMMARY

Care protocols share many similarities with clinical guidelines and integrated care pathways, and there are many linkages between the three. However, there are also differences between them and the terms are not synonymous. Care protocols tend to be more succinct than clinical guidelines, and integrated care pathways differ from care protocols in that they relate to individual patients' journeys. Although they may be based on and contain within them clinical guidelines or care protocols, they also include an evaluation of individual patients' responses.

Like clinical guidelines, care protocols should be developed in accordance with the current best evidence. As they are often less detailed than clinical guidelines, the information which supports their development may not be contained in the protocol itself, but should nonetheless be available to practitioners, and the quality of care protocols should be ascertained prior to using them. Care protocols may be perceived to carry a greater degree of obligation to adhere to them than clinical guidelines. However, like clinical guidelines, they should be used by individual practitioners in conjunction with their professional judgement, not unthinkingly applied in all situations.

Good-quality care protocols can be valuable in providing practitioners with summaries of evidence which they can use to initiate care rapidly, efficiently and effectively. However, they will only aid high-quality care provision if they are themselves of high quality and are appropriately used within the context of holistic care provision for individual patients. They may also improve the consistency of care provision, but will only achieve this if all the individuals or organisations involved in a patient's care are using the same protocol.

Using care protocols thus has the potential to improve the quality of care, in relation to both single procedures and entire care experiences. However, this is dependent on staff having the skills and knowledge needed to provide holistic care which links the aspects that are directed by protocols, and to use their judgement to determine when protocols are appropriate and when they should be modified or overridden.

5

Developing Clinical Guidelines and Care Protocols

Clinical guidelines and care protocols are intended to provide practitioners with applied summaries of the current best evidence regarding the clinical efficacy and cost-effectiveness of aspects of healthcare (DoH, 1998; Modernisation Agency and NICE, 2004a; Considine and Hood, 2000; Thomas, 1999). For them to achieve this, they must be developed in a way which ensures that the current best evidence is used, and that this is appropriately evaluated, summarised and synthesised. It must also be presented in a way that makes its application to practice clear. Those seeking to develop clinical guidelines or care protocols must therefore consider how they can achieve this, and those intending to use the guidance presented should know what constitutes a good standard of clinical guideline or care protocol, so as to be able to determine whether the guidance which they are considering using is of sufficient quality. This means being aware of the processes involved in clinical guideline development and the factors which are thought to indicate the quality of clinical guidelines and care protocols.

Clinical guidelines should be developed systematically (Considine and Hood, 2000). The process of guideline development should therefore include systematically gathering evidence, deciding on its quality, seeing how all the evidence fits together and from this forming conclusions about its application to practice settings. The conclusions from this process must then be presented in a way that is comprehensible and user-friendly. This chapter describes the main stages involved in the development of clinical guidelines and care protocols. Chapter 6 will discuss the quality indicators of clinical guidelines. Chapters 3 and 4 discussed what clinical guidelines and care protocols are and some of the differences between them. Notwithstanding these distinctions, the processes involved in developing clinical guidelines and care protocols have many similarities. In this chapter, the term 'clinical guideline' will generally be used for convenience, but the processes apply equally to developing care protocols or clinical guidelines where no distinction is stated.

Clinical Guidelines and Care Protocols

CHOOSING A SUBJECT

The first stage of the guideline development process is to identify that a guideline is necessary. This includes identifying that there is a need for information regarding an area of practice, deciding if this is a priority in comparison to other demands and determining whether the nature of the aspect of care in question means that a clinical guideline or care protocol is the best way to convey information about it.

In any area of practice, there are likely to be a number of aspects of care that would benefit from guidance being developed. However, it is unlikely to be feasible for individual wards or teams to concurrently develop guidelines respecting a large number of aspects of care. For example, on a paediatric medical unit it might be desirable to have clinical guidelines on the care of an infant with bronchiolitis, an infant or child with croup, a child with meningococcal disease, a child with meningitis, a child with diabetic ketoacidosis, a child with epilepsy a child with acute asthma. However, for many paediatric units, the resources required to simultaneously develop clinical guidelines in all these areas mean that it would not be feasible to do so. Decisions must therefore often be made as to which aspects of care have the highest priority or greatest urgency for guidance to be developed at any given time.

As a part of deciding which areas of practice have the greatest urgency for clinical guideline development, it is expedient to ascertain whether there are any existing guidelines or guidelines in the process of development that could be adopted, or adopted with modifications. This will avoid any unnecessary replication of work and will assist in making the best use of time and other resources. Nationally, the aim to avoid replication of work is one reason why NICE and SIGN work in close collaboration (SIGN, 2005).

If a clinical guideline regarding an area of practice already exists, a decision must still be made about whether or not to use it. The decision over whether or not to adopt an existing clinical guideline includes considering whether it is from or relates to an area which is the same or similar enough to the area to which its transfer is proposed for it to be applicable. For example, the national guideline on diabetic footcare (NICE, 2004f) could probably be used for the majority of the population of diabetics. However, a guideline on prone positioning of a critically ill adult might in part be transferable to a paediatric intensive care environment, but would be likely to require significant modification including the reasons for prone positioning, risk factors, staffing considerations and physiological parameters. In other cases, a guideline might be developed in the acute care setting which is not transferable to primary-care settings. For example, it has been suggested that the Royal College's guidance on chaperoning during intimate examinations requires some modification to be applicable to the primary-care setting (Rosenthal *et al.*, 2005). A decision must therefore be made regarding whether an existing guideline can be adopted as it stands, whether it can be adopted with modifications or whether it should not be adopted.

If there are a range of aspects of practice in which the development of clinical guidelines would be beneficial, and for which existing guidelines cannot be adopted, the priority of developing guidance for each area must be decided. This includes the urgency of the issue in question and the organisation's ability to support the workload of guideline development and implementation. These decisions will be influenced by a number of factors, including whether developing guidance fits with local and national targets or directives, whether it arises from audit data that reveal areas of specific concern, whether audit data can be used to assist in identifying the relative urgency of each area in which developing guidance might be useful, whether there have been any adverse incidents in practice, the recurrence of which might be avoided by having guidance available, and staff interests in and awareness of areas in which practice could be improved. There is no single correct way to decide on the priorities which direct guideline development, but, as Chapter 7 will discuss, the reason why clinical guidelines are developed and introduced into practice may affect their acceptance and the ease with which they can be implemented. The effort required to develop or adapt a clinical guideline will be wasted if it is not used, and thus organisational readiness for guideline use as well as the intrinsic value of a specific clinical guideline should be a strong consideration.

It is also important to consider whether or not a given aspect of care is compatible with the use of a clinical guideline or care protocol. There is a great deal more to healthcare provision than following guidelines or protocols, and, even if an aspect of care requires improvement or development, it does not necessarily follow that developing a clinical guideline or care protocol is the right way to achieve this. The aim of developing a clinical guideline or care protocol is to make a series of recommendations that can be widely generalised. Where the subject in question is not suitable for making such generalisations, it may well not be suitable for clinical guideline or care protocol development. Chapters 8 and 9 will discuss the importance of seeing guidelines or care protocols as a part, and not the totality, of the information which directs care. Deciding that a specific area of care is not appropriate for clinical guideline or care protocol development does not mean it is unimportant, only that it is not suitable for description in this type of document.

For example, if a problem is highlighted concerning the way in which midwives communicate with the women for whom they care, this is unlikely to be resolved by developing a clinical guideline or care protocol on the subject. The main aspects of communication which women consider to be important may be highlighted in guidelines, for example about how to organise maternity services so as to improve communication, the importance of giving women adequate time, privacy and a supportive environment and ascertaining their preferences and concerns. However, qualitative aspects of communication such as tone of voice and demeanour are personal attributes or skills that cannot be prescribed.

We have all probably experienced the irritation of being wished a 'nice day' by employees at fast-food outlets and other retail establishments, in a manner which clearly indicates that the last thing they care about is the quality of our day. 'Have a nice day' in this context really means 'Now take your change and get out of my way so I can serve the next customer'. However, its widespread and quasi insulting use seems to have developed from a protocol which was devised to make staff be friendly, show an interest in customers and thus improve sales. It is a communication protocol which has spectacularly failed to improve communication. Instead, it has produced a new irritation for us all to endure in the name of customer services. Or, if we view it in a more positive light (because I like to view the world in this vein), a child-friendly phrase to shout at drivers who cut us up at traffic junctions, and other people who annoy us beyond measure and whom we like to pointlessly insult out of their hearing, from cars and after slamming down phones.

The decision on whether or not to develop guidelines or care protocols includes considering not only the subject but also what the focus of the subject in question will be and why the guidance is needed. If a problem has been identified with communication between midwives and women whose first language is not English, the precise focus of the problem needs to be identified before a decision can be taken as to whether a clinical guideline or care protocol would be beneficial. If the problem is that midwives are aware of these deficits and would like to address them but are often unsure of how to access printed or recorded information in other languages and how to contact and organise translation services, a protocol for how to do this may be useful. However, if the problem is that midwives are unwilling to make the effort required to communicate effectively with individuals whose first language is not English, their attitudes are not very likely to be improved by the development of a protocol. Similarly, if the problem is found to be that staff in the area in question have generally poor communication skills, a protocol or guideline is unlikely to be successful in changing this. In these last two cases, educative discussion of the attitudes which lead to this situation is more likely to be effective in improving care.

In the case of national guidelines, there are set processes and criteria that direct how decisions will be made about the areas in which guidance will be developed. In England and Wales, guideline topics are referred to NICE by the Secretary of State for Health and the Welsh Assembly. Initial suggestions by individuals or organisations can also be made to NICE. The Advisory Committee on Topic Selection then assess each topic against set selection criteria. The committee membership includes representatives from the NHS, patient and carer groups, professional groups, the healthcare industry and specialist advisors. The Joint Planning Group (a group of senior staff from the DoH,

Welsh Assembly and NICE) then consider topics selected by the Advisory Committee for Topic Selection to check them against NICE's capacity to develop guidance, their technical feasibility and the best method(s) for developing guidance. Government health ministers then consider advice from the Advisory Committee for Topic Selection and the Joint Planning Group and decide which topics should be referred to NICE for guideline development.

The criteria which are used to select which topics are suitable for national guideline development are:

Whether this would promote the best possible improvement in patient care given the available resources

To achieve this, the proposed guidance must meet one or more of the following criteria:

- relate to an NHS clinical priority area, or to other government health-related priorities;
- address a condition that is associated with significant disability, morbidity or mortality in the population as a whole or in particular subgroups;
- relate to intervention(s) that could significantly improve patients' or carers' quality of life and/or reduce avoidable morbidity or premature mortality;
- relate to one or more interventions which, if used more extensively, would impact significantly on NHS or other societal resources;
- relate to an intervention(s) which could be used more selectively, without adversely affecting patient care, thus freeing up resources for use elsewhere in the NHS.

Whether NICE would be able to add value by issuing guidance

This includes considering whether the available evidence is sufficient to develop robust guidance and if there is evidence and/or reason to believe that there is or will be inappropriate practice and/or significant variation in clinical practice and/or variation in access to treatment (for example between geographical areas or social groups) if guidance is not issued.

Whether the most appropriate form of guidance consists of an appraisal, a clinical guideline or a combination of the two

This also takes into account whether there is any existing authoritative guidance on the subject, and the degree of urgency for guidance on any specific intervention.

For new interventions, whether the best option is to issue guidance at the time of launch of the intervention or at some specified future date

This takes into account:

- the possible impact of an absence of guidance at time of launch;
- the likely robustness of the evidence available at time of launch;
- the prospect of relevant additional data becoming available in the period immediately after the launch;
- whether safety and efficacy have already been assessed (or will be assessed in the near future) by the Interventional Procedures Advisory Committee (NICE, 2004j).

In Scotland, healthcare professionals and members of the public can suggest topics to SIGN. SIGN has seven speciality subgroups: cancer, cardiovascular disease, general medicine, mental health, primary care, surgery, and women's and children's health. Proposals for guideline development are given to the appropriate subgroup for consideration. The subgroup then seeks input from established clinical networks to identify their perceptions of the need for guidance. The speciality subgroups then submit a list of potential guideline topics to the Guideline Programme Advisory Group. This group select a limited number of proposals for discussion at the annual topic selection meeting of the SIGN council. They also consider how the suggested topics link with the work of NICE, so as to avoid replication.

SIGN's (2005) topic selection criteria are:

- the area is one of medical uncertainty, with evidence of wide variations in practice or outcome;
- the suggested area relates to conditions where there is proof that effective treatment exists and where mortality or morbidity can be reduced;
- the suggested area deals with iatrogenic diseases or interventions that carry significant risk or cost;
- the proposed guidance relates to a clinical priority area in the NHS in Scotland (the strategic aims for the NHS in Scotland are also considered in selecting topics);
- there is a perceived need for a guideline as indicated by the views of a network of relevant stakeholders.

ESTABLISHING PARAMETERS

Having decided to develop a clinical guideline or care protocol, the exact remit and parameters of the guidance need to be established (National Health and Medical Research Council, 2000; NHS Modernisation Agency and NICE,

2004b). The precise focus and limits of each clinical guideline should be decided and refined so that they are within manageable limits and to avoid attempting to include such a range of areas that the process of guideline development becomes unmanageable (Hughes, 2002). If the guideline development process becomes lengthy and convoluted, motivation amongst the development team may dwindle or the work be difficult to manage or too daunting for individuals to take on. Establishing clear parameters for a clinical guideline will increase the likelihood of its development being achieved and completed as promptly as possible. Clinical guidelines should be based on the current best evidence, but, if the time taken to develop them is excessive, there is a risk that they will be outdated almost before they are completed. Trying to develop guidance with too wide a remit also has the potential to create an unwieldy document that practitioners are unlikely to use. Chapter 7 will explore how guideline use can be enhanced, but it is important to bear in mind that, if guideline documents are not user-friendly and practitioners have to wade through a large and cumbersome document to find the information which they require, compliance is likely to be decreased. In some cases, it may be appropriate to attempt to cover a wide spectrum of issues in one guideline. For example, the NICE guideline on routine antenatal care (NICE, 2003d) includes the entire spectrum of care. In such cases, decisions must be made on how the work of guideline development will be made manageable for the guideline development team, for example by deciding very early on how the work will be divided into sections for small groups to take on, and how the end product will be made user-friendly and cohesive.

Having a focused clinical guideline includes providing a title which accurately reflects the content, to enable individuals who plan to use it to rapidly identify whether it is applicable to the care situations in which they are involved. The title of a guideline should therefore make clear exactly what is included in it and its limits as well as inclusions. A clinical guideline on pain management should make clear the situations in which the guideline is deemed to be applicable. This may include the age group and conditions that affect the applicability of the guideline's recommendations. For example, it might be that a guideline is limited to the management of postoperative pain in children. In other cases, the guideline might specify the healthcare sector for which its use is recommended, for example the NICE guideline on dyspepsia clarifies in the title that this concerns managing adults with dyspepsia in primary-care settings (NICE, 2004b).

IDENTIFYING A MULTIDISCIPLINARY DEVELOPMENT GROUP

Clinical guidelines should be constructed with representation from as many parties as possible, including all the disciplines that will be involved in their use (Thomas, 1999). In most instances, patients are cared for by a variety of healthcare professionals and the practice of one group of staff is likely to impact on the care provided by others. For example, care provided by nurses in relation to nutrition may also impact on the work of dieticians, medical staff and physiotherapists. In some cases, different disciplines carry out the same elements of care, for example medical and nursing staff can perform intravenous cannulation; physiotherapists and nurses perform chest physiotherapy in intensive care. As one intention of national care protocols is to increase the range of staff who can provide care (DoH, 2000), ensuring that an appropriate multidisciplinary group is convened to develop such protocols is important.

In other situations, an aspect of care may be performed by nurses, but the best method of providing this may be most appropriately decided in conjunction with other healthcare professionals whose knowledge will be beneficial. For example, a guideline on reintroducing enteral feeds following gastric surgery may have input from dieticians, nurses and surgeons, although it is likely to be nurses who actually recommence feeding. Identifying a guideline development group that includes representatives from all the staff groups who are affected by its use is therefore necessary (National Health and Medical Research Council, 2000; Hughes, 2002).

Consumers, health-policy analysts and economists should be included in the development of guidance (NHS Modernisation Agency and NICE, 2004b; National Health and Medical Research Council, 2000). It is also helpful to have individuals who are familiar with the process of developing guidelines in the group (Hughes, 2002). The intention is to ensure that all perspectives are covered in the development of guidance.

Involving service users in decision-making is currently seen as important in the provision of quality care, and this applies equally to the process of developing care protocols and clinical guidelines as to other areas of healthcare (NHS Modernisation Agency and NICE, 2004b). Arguably, this is even more important in developing guidance which will be generalised across populations and has the potential to affect large numbers of care recipients than where only one patient is affected. Unless service users are involved, there may be aspects of guidance omitted which are important to service users, or the guidance developed, while technically good, may be something that service users would not accept or something that they would not be able to enact.

When I was pregnant, I received a huge range of advice, from professionals, friends and curious folk who feel that pregnancy is a valid reason to cross the road and give their unsubstantiated opinion on just about everything and tell you details of their own intimate anatomy that you would sooner not hear about. When real-life advisors took a break, I was able to wade through the rainforest of pregnancy-related paper that came my way. Amongst this advice was a leaflet from one of the many organisations which are funded to provide advice to pregnant women. It advised that, if I found I was becoming tired during my pregnancy, I should be sure to take an afternoon rest ('try to lie down for an hour or so') and ideally create a couple of other breaks from activity during the day. It depicted a lady in sensible maternity wear, reclining on a plump sofa, while her grinning husband administered tea and biscuits. Now, this is all very good advice and would have suited me admirably had I had the necessary ingredients. However, anyone who is working full-time and has not yet managed to procure one of those useful self-cleaning houses, which are also equipped with a device that cooks and serves up your food and then washes up, and who does not have a partner standing by waiting to make tea and biscuits is unlikely to be able to follow it. I suspect this may represent a great deal of women. Most irritatingly of all, amongst the pastel-coloured pictures was a plateful of what looked to be nice chocolatey cookies which your partner was meant to offer you as you reclined. Raising my hopes for those was harder to forgive than the rose-coloured advice on taking leisurely breaks. To stave off further disappointment and associated unnecessary stress, I refused to read any more booklets.

This was, I am pleased to say, not advertised as being a clinical guideline, and the information was factually probably very true, because it was endorsed by a highly respected professional organisation. However, it was unlikely to be particularly practical to a large number of women in the real world. The same may occur with clinical guidelines which recommend steps which are, in theory, very good but which people in the real world cannot follow or for whom the effort of following the guidance would outweigh any benefit.

Involvement of service users may be achieved by including patient representatives and consumer- or interest-group representatives in the guideline development team. Patients' Forum or Patients' Advisory and Liaison Services (PALS) can also be involved as they may be able to provide information on patient views. Patient complaints and analysis of user feedback, both positive and negative, may be a useful additional source of information which can be used.

All those whose views and expertise are necessary for guideline development should be represented. However, Pagliari and Grimshaw (2002) found that there was often a disparity in the level of participation in or influence exerted on the guideline development process between the groups involved. They identified that medical consultants had a significantly higher input than general practitioners, nurses and other professions allied to medicine. They therefore suggest that group membership should be numerically balanced to avoid dominance by those disciplines who are likely to be perceived or to perceive themselves to have higher power status. Nonetheless, they acknowledge that this must be considered alongside the aim of keeping groups to a manageable size. Too large a group is likely to mean that decisions are not reached and that, far from ensuring an equality of power, some individuals' views are unlikely to be voiced or heard. Convening a guideline development group therefore requires decisions to be reached over how all the relevant groups can be represented in appropriate numbers while retaining a manageable group size. Therefore, despite the importance of the range of individuals whose knowledge, skills and experience are relevant being represented in the guideline development process, appropriate levels of representation for the degree of expertise needed from or offered by each group may be more important than numerical parity.

It may be necessary to convene a large group to develop a guideline, and this may be made manageable by deciding the parts into which a guideline will be developed and forming subgroups to explore these. However, given the risk of guidelines becoming unwieldy and the potential for every individual to have a personal slant which they wish to add, decisions will need to be made over the remit of the guideline, who will contribute, how the process will be conducted and managed and mechanisms put in place to ensure that subgroup work remains on target and focused on what the group has decided should be the remit of the guidance. Strong leadership is likely to be needed to keep the guideline development process on track and manage the entire group and any subgroups. This, as well as subject expertise, and often rather than subject expertise, may dictate who leads the guideline development process.

At a national level, the Bristol Inquiry (Kennedy, 2001) indicated that NICE must include input from across the healthcare professions and other interested parties in developing their guidance. NICE's NCCs receive representation from a number of relevant disciplines (NICE, 2005). For example, the NCC for Mental Health have a reference group which includes representation from the British Psychological Society, the Centre for Evidence-based Mental Health, the Centre for the Economics of Mental Health, the College of Occupational Therapists, the Institute of Psychiatry, the Manic Depression Fellowship, MIND, the National Institute of Social Work, Rethink Severe Mental Illness, the Royal College of General Practitioners, the Royal College of Nursing, the Royal College of Psychiatrists and the Royal Pharmaceutical Society. Once a topic is received for guideline development, the NCC establish guideline development groups for each guideline. These groups include health professionals, lay representatives and technical experts. This group develops a draft guideline on which registered stakeholders have two opportunities to comment. The guideline is also posted on the NICE website for comments during the consultation period. The Guideline Review Panel then review the guideline and checks that comments have been addressed.

In SIGN, guideline development is carried out by multidisciplinary groups who are intended to be nationally representative. The SIGN executive discuss with the topic proposer(s) and the appropriate specialty subgroup(s) and SIGN council which groups should be included in the guideline development group. SIGN guideline development groups vary in size depending on the scope of the topic under consideration, but generally comprise between 15 and 25 members, with the acknowledgement that there usually needs to be a trade-off between adequate representation of interested parties and achieving the optimum group size for effective decision-making. Patients and carers are involved in SIGN guideline development in three ways: through the literature search, through patient organisations and by ascertaining whether any other NHS groups are aware of additional information on patient views. SIGN also seek direct feedback from service users. SIGN have one national open meeting for commentary on each guideline that they develop, which anyone can attend. Guidelines are also subject to peer review by independent experts and lay reviewers (SIGN, 2005).

SEARCHING FOR EVIDENCE

Clinical guidelines should be developed from a systematic evaluation of the best available evidence (Considine and Hood, 2000; NICE, 2004). A major element of developing guidelines is therefore searching for and evaluating evidence. Having clear guideline parameters at the outset will make collecting evidence more manageable and focused. It is almost inevitable that some extraneous information will be gathered, but having a clear focus will assist to minimise this.

How evidence will be collected and how the tasks associated with collecting evidence will be divided amongst the guideline development group must be decided. Although evaluating and rating evidence is a separate part of the guideline development process, it will assist in information gathering if the group has a consensus on what types of evidence they consider appropriate from the start. Chapter 2 discussed what may be considered to constitute evidence. This includes research, papers based on physiological principles, case studies, expert opinion and patient experience (Rycroft-Malone, 2001). All these forms of evidence may be seen by the guideline development group as relevant; however, if the group aim to only accept papers which report RCT, it will be useful to decide this early on so as to increase the efficiency of searching.

Search criteria must also be decided. For example, if the group consensus is that only evidence from the past five years should be considered, it will allow all group members to limit their search to this time and ensure that only up-to-date information is used. If the group consensus is that, despite their possible value, non-English-language papers cannot be used as the group does not have the funding or language skills to translate them, these can be excluded from searches. This will again reduce the time wasted on obtaining information that will not be used and increase the consistency of searching between group members. The guideline group may decide that everyone will search for information across the board, or may divide the work into these subsections. In the latter case, consensus on search terms will relate to the subgroups considering each aspect of the guideline. For example, if a guideline is being developed on the administration of botulinum toxin for the treatment of muscle spasm in cerebral palsy, the guideline may include assessment of need, dose, frequency of administration, evaluation of effectiveness, possible side effects, actions to be taken and giving information to patients. Whether all of the group will address all these or divide them into subgroups should be decided. Clarifying search terms may also assist in ensuring that all aspects of the guideline will be covered and that only information that is relevant to the areas being covered is obtained.

How information will be sought should also be agreed, for example the databases to be used, additional resources to be included and how grey literature will be identified and used. This latter type of evidence is unpublished material such as theses and conference proceedings which will not appear on most searches but which may still be important evidence. It is often the most difficult to find, but its value should not be underestimated as it may be the most up-to-date information. Its use may therefore prevent a guideline becoming outdated or superseded by evidence that emerges soon after the guideline is published. If new evidence on the best way to manage aggression in autistic children has just been recorded in a PhD thesis, producing a guideline which does not include this would be unfortunate as it is likely that the work would soon be published and the guidance which was developed without it superseded.

APPRAISING AND SYNTHESISING EVIDENCE

Having obtained the evidence which will be used to develop a guideline, decisions must be made regarding how it will be appraised and synthesised. This includes developing a hierarchy of the relative importance which will be attributed to each form of evidence, developing or adopting a tool or tools to evaluate each piece of evidence and deciding how the review of evidence will be conducted (Hughes, 2002).

A variety of factors must be taken into account when deciding what types of evidence will be included in the final guideline, which evidence will be seen as carrying the greatest weight and how the quality of individual pieces of evidence will be assessed (CRD, 2001; Cochrane Collaboration, 2005; Hewitt-Taylor, 2003). As Chapter 2 identified, the decision over what is the best type of evidence should, first and foremost, be based upon the type of evidence which would be best for identifying facts about the subject in question, for example whether positivist or naturalistic research would be more appropriate and within this what methods would be the highest ranking. Where positivist research is seen as the best source of evidence RCTs will usually be seen as the highest form of evidence. However, although this may be seen as the highest form of evidence, the reality of guideline development may also be tempered by the ideal form of evidence being in scarce supply. Where there are relatively few RCTs in a given area, or where these are carried out on small groups of participants making the findings statistically insignificant, the data generated by this means may need to be augmented by data from other sources, such as case studies and expert opinion. The types of evidence available and the quality of the evidence will affect the strength of the recommendations made. Where the evidence in high-ranking categories of evidence is strong, for example where a number of high-quality, large randomised trials have been performed respecting a drug, and statistical significance achieved which clearly and unequivocally show what should be done, it will be easy to decide what to recommend. However, where only small studies exist which achieve borderline statistical significance, the relative importance of these in comparison with expert views or case studies will be less easy to precisely state, and recommendations will be less easy to make and will be less definite. Generally, the quality of evidence and the strength of recommendations are indicated on guidelines. For example, the SIGN guideline on management of childhood obesity indicates for each statement the level of evidence that informed it and for each recommendation the grade or strength with which it was made (SIGN, 2003a). This allows those using guidelines to know how good the evidence on which they are acting is and to incorporate this in discussions with patients.

Decisions must be made not only as to the relative importance which will be assigned to each form of evidence but also as to how the quality of studies will be decided, how differences in the findings between studies or disparities in the views of experts will be managed and how conclusions will be drawn.

The way in which the quality of individual pieces of evidence will be determined must be agreed. Guidance on evaluating research exists and can be used to direct the appraisal of a study's quality (CRD, 2001; Cochrane Collaboration, 2005). However, this tends to concentrate on positivist research, and in particular on RCTs. A blanket approach to evaluating qualitative research is not as easy to prescribe as the study designs used vary considerably, but a variety of tools exist which are suitable for evaluating research from the naturalistic paradigm (De Poy and Gitlin, 1994; Lincoln and Guba, 1986; Popay *et al.*, 1998). Although the focus on evaluation tools for positivist research in documents about clinical guidelines is possibly appropriate, as generalisability is usually their aim, positivist criteria should not be used to evaluate naturalistic studies.

More than one reviewer should assess each study, and a comparison of their views should be made to ensure that the guidance given represents a consensual view on the evidence and decrease the risk of bias or errors of judgement affecting the recommendations made. It is normal practice to develop rating scales to score evidence in systematic reviews, and a similar approach can be taken in developing guidelines. This will, as far as possible, ensure that the same things are being assessed by each reviewer and enable easy comparisons to be made between reviewers regarding a study's quality and the strength of its findings.

Cost must also be considered when guidance is being developed, and how cost is assessed is discussed in more detail in Chapter 10. The cost of an intervention should include how the apparent cost of providing an intervention compares with the potential reduction in costs of altered clinical outcomes if the intervention is given. NICE have made clear that, while it is not intended to be the overriding factor in healthcare decisions, cost is an important consideration in their recommendations for practice (Rawlins *et al.*, 2001). NICE include cost-effectiveness analysis in all their recommendations and undertake a cost-impact analysis for each guideline. SIGN do not undertake economic analysis but do include any relevant high-quality, published economic evaluation in the evidence, which they use to make a commentary on the resource implications of their recommendations if these are significant.

It is often neither possible nor desirable to pre-specify where cost will be placed in the hierarchy of evidence, as the importance of cost is dependent upon the strength of other forms of evidence and the amount of difference in cost between different interventions. The difference in cost between a new drug and an existing drug may be significant, but, if strong evidence of benefit from the new drug exists, cost may be less important than if the benefits are borderline. If the evidence of benefit from an intervention is very clear, and additional costs are minimal, cost may be unimportant. However, if the evidence of benefit is marginal and the cost high, cost is likely to be more important. Cost should also include cost of the intervention and associated costs, such as equipment and resources needed and staff time.

To return to my non-evidence-based flight booking from Chapter 1, I mostly look at the cost of flights because the rest of the information on the relative merits of an airline is not significant enough to influence me. However, if there were strong evidence that one airline had a propensity to land in the ocean, or to overbook so scandalously that at least 50% of passengers were usually turned away without decent compensation, I might move cost lower in my hierarchy of evidence. However, as all other things are more or less equal from my point of view, cost is a high priority, and usually top of my hierarchy of evidence. Although cost is my main concern in booking air transport, if a change of planes is required, the length of time that I will spend amusing a would-be toddler in an airport departure lounge is becoming an increasingly important feature. When he is old enough to want to pass the intervening hours spending money on toys and sweets in duty-free shops, it is something that will have to be included in the cost (indirect but potentially massive) category.

As well as the complexity of estimating the cost over time of non-intervention versus the cost of intervention, what constitutes a good outcome, who decides what a good outcome is and who assesses the cost must be decided. One of my best ever cost-benefit flights was a cheap deal from Los Angeles to Auckland. We, and about half the other backpackers checking in, were bumped off the flight. However, we were given $400 each (which more than covered our fare) and a night in the LAX Hilton. When you have been back-packing for five months and just driven 400 km or so from Death Valley to LA, $400 and a night in the LAX Hilton instead of a night flight to New Zealand (when you are guaranteed to get a flight the next day and have nothing special planned except six weeks' hiking) is a very good outcome. You can also stock up on those sachets of soap, shampoo and moisturiser and get a new little sewing kit. However, for a businessperson who has meetings the next day and who has spent many nights in hotels and who is well provisioned with sachets of goodies and sewing kits, the outcome might be seen very differently. So, whose view of a good outcome for the price being used is very important to decide. The airline knew this, and only backpackers were being asked to stand down. Everyone seemed to accept this. This was a few years ago and I suspect that the LAX Hilton has only just recovered from the mass of unwashed bodies and outbreak of low-key toiletries theft that it endured.

There is also some evidence that estimates of cost may be presented very differently by different groups, for example drug-company representatives and independent analysts have been reported to reach different conclusions about cost (Miners *et al.*, 2004). When cost is being evaluated, the quality and origin of the evidence on cost must therefore be considered and how and by whom the cost-versus-benefit is to be decided determined.

INCORPORATING EXPERT OPINION

Expert opinion may be one of the forms of evidence that informs the development of guideline statements, but it should also be sought on emergent guidance (NHS Modernisation Agency and NICE 2004b). It is possible that experts in the field of practice will be able to identify some of the practical issues involved in the implementation of a guideline which an RCT or theoretical knowledge of the subject would not. The aim of guidance is for it to be used, and seeking the views of experts on emergent guidance may mean that any vagueness, practical flaws or aspects of the guidance which practitioners are not likely to understand or accept may be able to be identified and rectified.

Once the guideline has been designed, it should be reviewed by representatives from the range of interested disciplines. The aim of this step is to ascertain whether, on this evidence, they would produce similar recommendations, and whether other healthcare professionals would understand and apply the recommendations in a similar manner. The reviewers should not have been involved in the guideline development process, so that their views are more likely to be representative of how clinicians who receive the document will interpret and use it. The guideline should then be tested and evaluated in a selected healthcare setting (Thomas, 1999). Chapter 7 discusses the guideline implementation process, but implementing new guidance is time-consuming and therefore costly and its practicality should ideally be tested prior to expending time and effort in the widespread distribution and implementation of a document which may require modification because the instructions in it are unclear, ambiguous or not practical.

EVALUATION

Guideline development should include a strategy for any evaluation of the guideline (Max *et al.*, 2003). The evaluation strategy should include whether the guideline is used, but should also provide the opportunity to identify the reasons for non-use, if this is the case, and the effectiveness of the guideline in improving patient care. Chapter 6 deals in more detail with how to evaluate clinical guidelines, but an evaluation strategy should be devised at the time of designing clinical guidelines and should include more than simply whether the guideline was used or not.

UPDATING

Once clinical guidelines have been developed, they must be kept up to date (Aiello *et al.*, 2004). If guidance remains unchanged when new evidence emerges, it will not represent the current best evidence. Gartlehner *et al.* (2004) nonetheless identify that deciding when to update guidelines is not easy. The guideline development process is expensive and time-consuming. Very frequent updating of guidelines is likely to be expensive and impractical and makes guideline implementation difficult. However, infrequent updating means that guidelines are at risk of recommending ineffective, outdated or unsafe practice. At the design stage it is therefore important to decide how and when updating will occur.

As well as identifying a review date for guidelines, how emergent evidence will be identified and included before the review date occurs must be decided. New information is almost constantly emerging in healthcare, and it would be inadvisable for a guideline not to be amenable to alteration prior to the date set for review if evidence emerges which means that it should be altered. It is to be assumed that the majority of those involved in developing a guideline will have an interest in the subject and will be abreast of developments in the field, but the exact mechanisms for such updating should be decided at the outset.

IMPLEMENTATION

The intention of clinical guidelines and care protocols is that they should be used to influence practice. Chapter 7 discusses how the implementation of clinical guidelines and care protocols may be optimised, and the implementation stage should receive as much attention as the development of guidelines. Without implementation in practice, clinical guidelines and care protocols are of little value. Their intention is to improve practice, and this will not be achieved unless attention is given to how they will actually be used.

SUMMARY

The process of developing clinical guidelines should be systematic, and the final document should present guidance in a user-friendly format. Guideline development includes identifying areas in which guidance is needed, whether this area is suitable for a clinical guideline or care protocol to be developed, whether the development of a guideline or care protocol is a current organisational priority and whether the necessary resources are in place to enable guideline development and implementation to proceed.

Having decided that the development of a clinical guideline or care protocol is possible and appropriate, the exact remit of the guideline, its parameters and the way in which evidence will be gathered and synthesised must be decided. A multidisciplinary guideline development group should be convened, with representation from an appropriate range of disciplines and groups while simultaneously being of a manageable size.

Evidence should be systematically sought and evaluated, and the place which each type of evidence, including cost, will occupy in the guidance that is developed must be decided. The evidence which has been gathered and evaluated must then be presented in a clear and unambiguous format which healthcare professionals can easily follow in practice. The guidance which has been developed should be reviewed by independent experts prior to being used. It is expedient to carry out some form of piloting of any new guidance so as to avoid the costly and time-consuming implementation of clinical guidelines and care protocols to which adjustments will have to be made.

Guidelines should have a mechanism for evaluation both of their use and of the outcomes of their use. They should have a date set for formal review and an agreed review mechanism for unscheduled updating in light of emergent evidence.

6

Using Clinical Guidelines and Care Protocols

The intention of clinical guidelines and care protocols is that they should facilitate the use of evidence in practice, and therefore equal effort should be devoted to the way in which guidelines and protocols are, or can be, used as is given to developing them. Unless they are used to improve practice, the efforts expended in developing guidance will be wasted. Chapter 7 will discuss the process of guideline implementation once a decision has been taken to use a clinical guideline or care protocol. This chapter will focus on how individuals and organisations can decide whether or not to use an existing clinical guideline or care protocol, and whether its ongoing use is appropriate.

The ways in which clinical guidelines and care protocols can be evaluated have many similarities, and therefore, as was the case in Chapter 5, for convenience, the term 'clinical guideline' is generally used in this chapter to refer to both clinical guidelines and care protocols.

Before a decision is taken to use an existing clinical guideline, its overall intrinsic quality and its applicability to the situation in which its use is proposed should be assessed. Assessing the quality of a clinical guideline or care protocol is easier and more likely to be accurate if there are criteria against which to evaluate it. The stages which were identified in Chapter 5 in relation to developing clinical guidelines and care protocols give some indication of the quality issues which should be considered. However, it is also useful to have a framework for assessing the quality of clinical guidelines.

The AGREE Collaboration (2001) have issued an instrument that provides a validated, internationally agreed framework which forms a good basis for evaluating the quality of clinical guidelines and care protocols, and this provides the structure for this chapter. In Chapter 5, it was suggested that the quality of the evidence used to develop guidance should be assessed by more than one reviewer to increase the accuracy and reliability of assessment and to guard against bias. The same principle applies to assessing the quality of an existing guideline, and the AGREE Collaboration (2001) suggest that a guideline should be assessed by at least two, and preferably four, assessors. They recommend that each aspect of the guideline should be rated on a four-point scale ranging from 'strongly agree' (scores 4 points) to 'strongly disagree' (scores 1 point) that the criteria for quality has been met. However, they recommend that the scores from across domains should not be aggregated to give one overall score representing the quality of a guideline. Rather, they should be used to provide information on the strengths and weaknesses of the aspects which are assessed.

The domains of clinical guidelines which AGREE recommend should be evaluated are:

THE SCOPE AND PURPOSE OF THE GUIDELINE

The objectives and/or questions which are covered by the guideline and the patient groups to whom the guideline is meant to apply should be clear (AGREE, 2001).

As well as indicating the group to whom guidance applies, for example children with cystic fibrosis, patients who are undergoing liver transplantation and adults with a learning disability, clinical guidelines should include a clear indication of the range of aspects of the subject that they cover. In some cases, a clinical guideline will cover all aspects of a subject, but in others it will not. For example, NICE (2005c) have issued a guideline on lung cancer that covers the majority of aspects of care but have also developed a range of guidelines concerning diabetes which include separate, specific documents on type 1 diabetes (NICE, 2004g), type 2 diabetes blood-glucose management (NICE, 2002b), type 2 diabetes retinopathy (NICE, 2002e), type 2 diabetes renal disease (NICE, 2002d), type two diabetes management of blood pressure and blood lipids (NICE, 2002c) and type 2 diabetes footcare (NICE, 2004f).

As well as checking whether a guideline clearly states the population to which it applies and the aspects of their care that it covers, it is necessary to check that the guideline's content actually addresses these. A clinical guideline which claims, from its title, to be about the management of adults and children with major head injuries should include the management of adults and children and should focus on major head injuries. Although some mention of minor head injuries and their management may be necessary, for example in distinguishing the two, the main focus should be on major head injuries.

As well as the group of people to whom the guideline applies and the interventions or aspects of care which are covered, the objectives of a guideline should be clear (AGREE, 2001). Where possible, guidelines should therefore indicate what the expected outcome of their use is. This may be difficult to state, but having clarity over the objective of the guideline will assist practitioners to decide if it addresses the needs of the population for whom they care and any specific needs which have been identified in their area of practice. For instance, if staff on a surgical ward have identified that a higher-than-average number of patients on their ward develop wound infections, a guideline on postoperative care whose objectives included reduction in wound infection might be attractive. On the other hand, a guideline which omitted wound care, focusing instead on haemodynamic monitoring in the first 24 hours postoperatively might not be a priority for that ward to implement, regardless of its intrinsic value. Having clear objectives will also be helpful in ascertaining whether a guideline is effective in so far as it achieves what it sets out to achieve. For example, it may be that a guideline on infection control in hospitals intends to reduce the incidence of hospital-acquired infection by 20% within a year. This kind of aim will assist in any evaluation of the guideline's effectiveness as to whether or not this reduction is achieved and can be assessed. Later in this chapter, the ways in which clinical guidelines' effectiveness may be evaluated are discussed, and that they have clear objectives will assist in this.

The title of a clinical guideline should therefore be clear and unambiguous and state the content and limits of the guideline, and the guideline should include clear objectives.

STAKEHOLDER INVOLVEMENT

There should be evidence that clinical guidelines have been developed with involvement from appropriate professional groups, that patients' views and preferences were sought, that target users have been clearly defined and that piloting of the guideline has occurred (AGREE, 2001).

Appropriate Professional Representation

Clinical guidelines should include details of membership of the guideline development group, as this enables potential users to determine whether all the relevant perspectives appear to be represented. If the group which develops a clinical guideline on the postoperative management of patients following knee replacement, for example, includes orthopaedic surgeons, physiotherapists and nurses, it would be fair to assume that the entirety of postoperative management has been represented, and therefore the guidelines could be said to be valid. If the perspectives of all the major parties involved in a care situation are not represented, it is likely that the guideline will not include all professional perspectives and will have the potential to have missed important aspects of care, or to be unacceptable to some professional groups. This has the potential to impair not only the quality of care provided in accordance with such guidance but also the acceptability of the guidance to all staff groups.

As well as guidelines indicating whether the appropriate people were involved in its development, it should include the actions to be taken by all the relevant multidisciplinary team members. It will be somewhat counter-productive for a guideline on infant feeding to be used by nursing staff on a paediatric ward if dieticians are following a separate protocol and medical staff another. It will also be problematic if practice nurses are following one guide-line for managing asthma in primary care while GPs are following another. Thus, as well as multidisciplinary involvement in developing guidance, a good guideline will include multidisciplinary working in the guidance itself. A guide-line existing cannot, of course, of itself guarantee that it will be used by all team members, but if there is evidence of multidisciplinary involvement in its development and if it is worded so as to cover the roles of all the members of the multidisciplinary team, it is more likely to be used across the board and provide consistent care.

Patient Views

There should be evidence of patient representation in guideline development. If there is no evidence that patients' views were sought, it is possible that the guidance given, despite being technically 'correct', will not be acceptable to service users, or will not address the aspects of care which patients see as most important.

However well accepted evidence is by healthcare professionals, unless patients agree to treatment or care, this should not usually be instituted. Although the challenges inherent in implementing the recommendations made in clinical guidelines or care protocols are often discussed in relation to healthcare staff, patients' preferences and views will also affect their imple-mentation. There is a suggestion that one reason for good evidence not being used in practice is that it does not accord with patients' preferences (Ricart *et al.*, 2003; Flottorp and Oxman, 2003; Tracy *et al.*, 2003). Cultural issues and personal preferences may affect whether or not a guideline is acceptable to patients, even if it is technically good. For example, a guideline may recommend screening which is not acceptable to some social, ethnic or religious groups. Thus, when deciding whether or not to adopt a guideline, whether it will be acceptable to patients as well as staff is important. An indi-cation of the level of patient involvement in the guideline development process is a useful indicator of whether the guidance set out will be accept-able to patients.

Previous chapters have identified that clinical guidelines and care protocols can be used as a part of quality-assurance mechanisms. Whether or not service users view the guidance given as commensurate with quality care will give some indication of whether it will improve care from their perspective. A guideline may seem to healthcare staff to be likely to improve the quality of care, but if it does not include or address the aspects of care which patients see as important its use is unlikely to enhance the quality of care as perceived by them. If the intention of quality-measurement mechanisms is to assess whether patients receive quality care, their perspectives should be included in the standards by which quality will be assessed. As Chapter 5 identified, not all aspects of quality of care are amenable to the kind of information contained in a clinical guideline or care protocol. However, user involvement in guideline development will give some indication as to whether patients would consider that the points included in the guidance are commensurate with a good standard of care. For example, a clinical guideline on the care of adults who require long-term tracheostomy which did not include any indication of consideration of altered body image might address all the medical and technical aspects of care very comprehensively. However, it might leave a significant gap in what patients would see as quality care.

Piloting

Clinical guidelines and care protocols are intended to give information which improves the consistency as well as the quality of care. To achieve this, the guideline must be interpreted in the same way by all users. Whether this is likely to occur may be ascertained by asking a group which is representative of those who will be using the guideline to review it, or by piloting its use. A good guideline will include evidence that piloting has occurred, and, if a guideline does not include this, it is expedient for potential users to pilot it or check for consistency of interpretation prior to attempting any widespread implementation of it. Implementing new guidance is labour intensive and costly in terms of staff education, and changing practice. Whether the guidance being proposed is feasible in practice and whether or not the guideline document can be easily understood and used should therefore be determined before effort is expended and costs incurred in implementing the recommendations.

RIGOUR OF DEVELOPMENT

The rigour of the guideline development process should be assessed, including whether evidence was systematically collected and evaluated, whether the recommendations were developed rigorously and whether the links between the evidence and the recommendations are clear. Guidelines should be externally reviewed by experts, and a schedule for updating should be included (AGREE, 2001).

Systematic Searching

Clinical guidelines should be a valid summary of the current best evidence on the subject that they address. A guideline should provide details of the methods and the criteria that were used for searching for evidence so that potential users have a means of rapidly assessing the likely quality of the evidence that has been gathered.

Theoretically, those evaluating the guideline can themselves gather, evaluate and synthesise the available evidence and see if this matches that which has been used in the guideline. However, one of the reasons for clinical guidelines being developed is because it is unrealistic to expect every practitioner to seek out, appraise and collate all the evidence on every aspect of the care in which they are involved. Although individuals or groups can search for and appraise the evidence to determine whether a guideline includes this, doing so conflicts with the reason for adopting an 'off the peg' guideline as it means that a great deal of the work which would be required to develop a clinical guideline or care protocol oneself must be carried out. The reality is therefore that a significant number of practitioners will take a number of recommendations made in guidelines on trust. However, they should be able to gain some assurance that their trust is well placed.

A common-sense approach is therefore for those who are considering adopting a guideline to check the ways in which information was searched for and the criteria used to select this, so that a judgement can be made as to whether this seems likely to produce the best range of evidence. For instance, if relatively few databases were searched, the full range of information may not have been gathered. If grey literature had not been included, the guideline may become outdated more quickly than if it had been.

Methods Used for Formulating Recommendations

For a guideline to be of good quality, and to provide sound guidance for practice, all the relevant evidence must have been gathered, evaluated, interpreted correctly and the appropriate recommendations made. In order to truly establish whether a guideline has achieved this, it would be necessary to check whether all sources, or at least the principal ones used, have been accurately interpreted and that the guideline recommendations fit the evidence from which they are derived. As with seeking information, this would be time-consuming and defeat the object of adopting a ready-made guideline. Thus, having explicit details of how recommendations were made will be useful to enable guideline users to assess whether the processes followed to evaluate data and to make recommendations were appropriate and seem likely to result in sound recommendations being made.

AGREE (2001) suggest that there should be evidence that the health benefits, side effects and risks of the recommendations have been considered in clinical guideline development. If there is evidence that these criteria are achieved, it suggests that the process of guideline development was thorough and unbiased as the disadvantages and risks as well as the benefits of the recommended actions have been taken into account. For example, the issue of service-user representation in a guideline dealing, in part, with service-user feedback is important, for that feedback might be deemed inadequate if the sample of patients used does not sufficiently reflect the whole spectrum of service-users within healthcare.

External Review

A new clinical guideline should be reviewed by experts from appropriate disciplines prior to it being published, and guidelines should include information on the group who acted as reviewers. This provides further evidence that the guidance is considered by experts in the field, who do not have any vested interest in its development, to be an unbiased summary of the best available evidence. It should also contribute to there being a degree of confidence that the statements made in the guideline will be clear to users as a panel of experts have understood them to mean the same thing. In the same way that it is expedient to check that there is adequate representation from lay and professional groups in guideline development, it is expedient to check whether there is adequate representation from across groups in the review process.

Procedure for Updating

A clinical guideline will only facilitate care in accordance with the current best evidence if it is up to date. Guidelines should therefore indicate when they were developed, and also when they are scheduled for review. This allows users to determine whether they include up-to-date evidence. It also allows them to determine whether or not they should await an update of the current guidance before investing time and effort in introducing a new guideline in practice. It is likely to be counterproductive to expend time and effort in encouraging staff to change practice or follow a guideline if this will soon be superseded and they will have to become accustomed to another set of guidance, first, because it will waste valuable time and, secondly, because it may give the impression that it is not beneficial to change practice as this will only need to be changed again in the near future.

CLARITY AND PRESENTATION

The AGREE (2001) criteria include assessing the clarity with which guidance is presented. This comprises the recommendations made being clear and unambiguous, the key recommendations being easily identifiable and the inclusion of tools for the application of the guideline.

Clarity

Clinical guidelines should provide clear guidance so that practitioners can use them to provide care with confidence. In Chapters 3 and 4, the potential for clinical guidelines and care protocols to improve patient safety and reduce errors was discussed. However, this will only be the case if the guidance given is applied to practice, clear and unequivocal. If guidelines are unclear, staff either are unlikely to use them or, if they use them, may not follow them as intended and may therefore not provide optimum care, and may even provide unsafe or incorrect care. For example, a clinical guideline for administering intravenous fluids to a child with diabetic ketoacidosis must make clear whether any initial resuscitation bolus that is required is or is not included in the fluid replacement calculations for the next 48 hours. If this is not clear, there is a potential for staff to interpret the guidance given inconsistently. Perhaps more importantly, it means that fluid administration may be inaccurate, which may be harmful, particularly in small children. Guidelines which do not give clear statements about what should be done may also cause unnecessary and potentially dangerous delays in care provision while practitioners seek to decipher the meaning of the guidance. Thus, the guideline statements should leave practitioners in no doubt about what action they should take or the options which are recommended. For instance, a clinical guideline on the management of a patient immediately post myocardial infarction should present information on how to care for the patient, for example what monitoring is recommended and for how long, what drugs and other therapeutic interventions are recommended in each situation and how their effectiveness should be assessed, as well as the evidence to support this guidance. This should be presented in a logical sequence so that it can be followed step by step.

This point links with whether there is evidence that the guideline has been piloted, and whether experts in the field of practice have reviewed it, as these stages will allow some testing of whether the guideline is clear and unambiguous.

Additional Tools

Clinical guidelines are intended to be directly applicable to practice. However, because they also need to present the supporting evidence which will allow decisions to be made as to their quality, they may become somewhat cumbersome. It may then be difficult for practitioners to identify the key points, which they need to be able to do quickly. They may therefore benefit from including or being supported by clear step-by-step guides or flow charts or by including care protocols within clinical guidelines which summarise the main points made so as to provide quick reference guides for use in practice. For example, the NICE guideline on the initial management of head injuries includes four clinical practice algorithms (NICE, 2003g). Such summaries may be useful so that the recommended actions in given clinical situations can be rapidly identified and followed logically. There may also be supporting literature in the form of patient information leaflets or educational tools contained within clinical guidelines (SIGN, 2005). For example, the SIGN clinical guideline on childhood obesity includes a diagram and supporting information on the 'healthy plate' model, which can be used for patient and staff education (SIGN, 2003a).

The documentation provided with clinical guidelines may also include documents which can be used in conjunction with the guideline, such as patients' records where the stages which are recommended in a clinical guideline can be commented on, and evaluated, like those seen in integrated care pathways. Ideally, clinical guidelines should also include documentation which can be used for the collection of evaluative data on the guideline.

APPLICABILITY

AGREE include in their applicability criteria potential organisational barriers to guideline implementation and the cost of guideline development and implementation. They also state that review criteria should be included in the guidance.

Part of the decision over whether or not to adopt an existing clinical guideline is whether or not it can be used to inform practice as it stands, and whether it is applicable to the practice area in question. A guideline may be of high quality, but if it is applied in an inappropriate setting it will not enhance care. A guideline that is adopted by a clinical area should have been designed for use in a situation which is sufficiently similar for its transfer to be appropriate. Therefore, as well as the intrinsic quality of the guideline, its applicability to a given setting must be determined. This includes considerations such as the patient group to which its transfer is proposed, whether it was designed for use in primary- or secondary-care settings and its country of origin. For example, a guideline on management of violence in a hospital setting may not be directly transferable to the primary-care setting, and a guideline on establishing home 'Total Parenteral Nutrition' devised in the United States may require modification before being used in England because of the differences in referral pathways and titles and role remits of the healthcare professionals involved.

Potential Organisational Barriers to Implementation

Chapter 7 will discuss the issues involved in implementing clinical guidelines in practice, but decisions about whether or not to use a guideline include considering the organisation's readiness for the guideline to be used. This can include issues surrounding the readiness for change of individuals within the organisation, and any other significant changes which are currently underway or anticipated. While a disinclination to change is not a reason to avoid attempting to change practice, the readiness of individuals and concurrent changes being experienced will affect whether it is expedient to attempt to introduce a clinical guideline at any given point in time, and how this should be done. A clinical guideline may include details of the systems which should be in place to enable it to be implemented. These may include equipment, staffing and funding. It may be that changes which extend beyond the ward or Trust involved are needed to implement guidance, for example if recommendations are to be followed regarding the establishment of a nurse-led rheumatology service this will require cooperation from nurses, rheumatologists, Trust managers, GPs who refer patients, other professions, such as physiotherapists, and patients. How this will be achieved should be considered before guideline implementation is attempted.

If the appropriate support systems are not in place to allow successful guideline implementation and it is doomed to failure, there will be no benefit in it being introduced, however compelling the evidence that it might be beneficial. These considerations will have to be weighed against the problems which may result from non-use. However, if there is absolutely no chance that guidance can really be used, it is pointless to attempt this as it will either result in obvious failure or the adoption of new practice in name while the reality of practice remains unchanged.

More potentially problematic for individual practitioners is the question of when a guideline which has been adopted for use should not be used in individual cases. Chapter 8 discusses the balance between clinical guidelines and expertise in practice and the legal aspects of guideline use. However, one overriding theme in the use of clinical guidelines is that they are not intended to replace clinical judgement and should be used in conjunction with this and patient preferences. The salient point for clinical guideline use is that simply because a guideline exists and has been approved by an organisation, nationally such as the NICE or SIGN or locally for instance by an acute or primary-care Trust, does not mean that the guideline must be followed slavishly when this is not in the patient's best interests. Neither will this necessarily be defensible in law.

Cost

Clinical guidelines should take into account cost-effectiveness as well as clinical efficacy. Although, as discussed in Chapters 2 and 5, the relative importance of cost depends on the strength of other forms of evidence, and the degree of cost, it cannot be omitted from the evidence which is used to inform practice. Clinical guidelines should therefore give an indication of the estimated cost versus benefit of the recommendations which they make and, like other forms of evidence, state how conclusions about this were reached. The importance which the guideline developers attribute to cost and why this is the case should also be clear.

Local budgetary considerations may also be an issue in deciding whether or not an existing guideline can be used. For example, although the balance of clinical efficacy and cost-effectiveness over time may dictate a certain course of action, this may not be something which an NHS Trust can afford at a given point in time, or they may have inadequate funds for the necessary equipment or staff training to achieve this. Adopting a guideline in name which cannot be successfully implemented because of a lack of resources is not likely to be a helpful approach. It may, in such instances, be possible to adopt some parts of a guideline or to develop a strategy for achievement over a span of five years as funding allows with interim arrangements for addressing the elements of guidance which cannot be funded at this point in time.

Review Criteria

A good guideline should be able to be relied upon to produce a given result if it is used appropriately. However, this can only be identified when the effectiveness of the guideline is evaluated. Guidelines may include existing evaluative evidence as supporting information, such as how readmission rates have been affected by using a clinical guideline for the care of children with febrile seizures, or how cost-effectiveness has been improved by using a guideline on the management of abdominal pain in adults in accident and emergency departments. Such information will not always be available, particularly with relatively new guidelines, but it is essential that a method of evaluating whether or not guidelines make a difference to patient care exists. A good clinical guideline should therefore include clear evaluative criteria. If it does not, evaluative criteria must be developed so that its reliability in achieving the desired outcomes can be evaluated. Evaluation of a guideline should include whether or not it is used, if it contributes positively to care and its cost.

The mechanism for auditing or evaluating a guideline should include whether or not the guideline is used and, if not, the reason for this. It is of little benefit to continue to produce a clinical guideline and to educate staff in its use if it is not subsequently used in practice. If a guideline is not used, it is important to know why this is the case so that this can be addressed. For instance, staff may not be aware that the guideline exists, the guideline may need to be modified to make it more user-friendly or practical or, if it is inappropriate and this is the reason for non-usage, it may need to be withdrawn.

The fact that a guideline exists and is thought to have been implemented in a given area does not provide any guarantee that staff are using it. Livesey (2005) found that compliance with a multiagency protocol for managing sudden and unexpected infant and childhood death was poor despite the protocol having supposedly been endorsed by staff and implemented in practice.

A method of evaluating whether guidelines are actually used, not just whether individuals or organisations claim to use them, is therefore necessary. Establishing whether a clinical guideline which is ostensibly in use is actually used is not easy. Self-report is one option. However, self-report can be problematic and its accuracy is dependent, amongst other things, on whether or not staff feel able to admit to not using a guideline. Anonymity in self-reporting may assist in this, as may assurances regarding the purpose of checking whether guidelines are being used and clarification that punitive action will not be taken against those not complying, provided this is the case. However, this may not be enough to guarantee honesty. One of the anecdotes which crops up from time to time in higher education is of a faculty which was asked to provide an anonymous self-report of teaching time so that an estimate of the total number of teaching hours needed by the faculty could be made. The legend is that the results of the anonymous self-report detailed just over twice as many hours teaching as would be available if every faculty member worked ten hours a day, 365 days a year. Someone, somewhere, was exaggerating.

Observation may be used but will be difficult to effect in many cases, and costly. It may be more realistic to carry out audits at preset intervals or to audit charts or patients' records if these give an indication of whether or not guidelines were used. However, this, like self-report, may be flawed, especially if staff follow some but not all aspects of a guideline or protocol, or if, in a significant number of cases, documentation is absent. It may be that a specific evaluative study can be set up alongside the implementation of a new guideline so that observation, self-report and the audit of notes can be combined to allow a triangulation of data. However, this is unlikely to be possible in many cases, or for a prolonged time.

Auditing the use of guidelines will show if they are used but will not provide data on whether this makes a difference to patient care. Evaluation tools should therefore include a mechanism for evaluating how far clinical guidelines contribute to the quality of care provision. The fact that a clinical guideline or care protocol is used cannot be assumed to mean that this is advantageous, even if the evidence upon which the guideline is predicated indicates that this should be the case. It may increase cost, reduce the standard of care received or be harmful to patients. An evaluation of a guideline therefore requires there to be clarity over the intention of the guideline, how success will be measured or demonstrated and what is the most important outcome, for example improved cost-effectiveness, improved physiological parameters or improved overall quality of life as perceived by patients. A range of outcomes may be deemed to be equally important, and the evaluative criteria will depend upon the nature of the guideline and its main aims. They may therefore need to include quantitative and qualitative data and to incorporate ways of ascertaining information on long-term and short-term clinical outcomes and the views of staff and patients.

Physiological parameters may be used to assess the effectiveness of clinical guideline use, for example, if a guideline on diabetic care is being used, it may be appropriate to assess whether the blood-sugar levels of those using the guideline are more stable than either those who are not or in comparison to the same patients before guideline use. Sometimes pre- and post-guideline-use comparisons will be problematic as pre-guideline data may not be available. In some instances, patients will have been recording physiological parameters prior to the use of new guidance or these may be available in their health records, but this will not always be the case. Where pre-and post-guideline data are not available, it may still be possible to determine whether using the guidance seems to produce reasonable results and is safe, for example that patients using a new clinical guideline for diabetic care achieve adequate blood-sugar control. There may of course be an artefactual effect in so far as focusing more on their diabetes because of having a new guideline to follow may produce better compliance in some patients. Whether this matters or not is arguable. If having the clinical guideline, rather than following it, produces a positive effect may not be important clinically, as the patient's health is still improved, but it does not validate the guideline itself and the effect may not be sustained after the initial novelty value of the guideline wears off. This type of initial improvement followed by deterioration or return to baseline should be considered in planning the timing, frequency and duration of evaluation.

Admission and readmission rates and mortality statistics may also be used to evaluate the effect of using clinical guidelines. These may, however, have the problem of confounding variables, and the time before the effect of a guideline would be seen should be considered. For example, it might be some time before the use of a guideline on coronary heart disease prevention showed actual effects on morbidity and mortality. In contrast, a guideline on the management of acute asthma in accident and emergency departments might be expected to show more immediate improvements in data, such as length of admission and mortality.

When and how often the effect of a clinical guideline should be evaluated will depend upon what is being assessed. This should be planned alongside the introduction of the guideline so that a logical pattern and pathway is followed and all parties are clear over when and how they can expect to see or know about the effectiveness of a guideline. All the elements of the evaluation of a clinical guideline may not be able to be assessed at the same time, for example the financial benefit of a new drug being used to treat migraine may need to be assessed over a year, whereas patients' reports on the extent to which this drug controls their symptoms may be available within a few months.

The time taken for guidelines to be used effectively, as well as the time taken for them to produce results, must also be taken into account when designing the evaluation framework so that the evaluation measures actual, and not supposed, practice. Using a clinical guideline on endotracheal suctioning which recommends the use of closed-suction systems might initially indicate that closed systems are more costly because of staff discarding systems earlier than they should or using them incorrectly, or because of initial outlay costs. As staff become used to the new approach, savings may become apparent and the timing and duration of evaluation should take this into account. Evaluation which occurs before a guideline is in regular use or being used correctly will not be a reliable method of evaluating its effectiveness. All other aspects of guideline evaluation should therefore be matched against whether or not a guideline is actually being used. For example, if there appears to be no cost benefit following guideline implementation, it is important to know whether this is because there is no saving or because the guideline was seldom adhered to or adhered to in part but not in whole.

How patient satisfaction can be measured will depend upon the population being studied, and the aspect of satisfaction which is being explored. It may be appropriate to issue quantitative questionnaires, for example to identify whether using a guideline on the management of angina reduces the number and intensity of episodes of chest pain which patients experience. In other cases, it may be more appropriate to use qualitative approaches, for example for exploring the experiences of autistic children's parents of their child's hospitalisation following the introduction of a clinical guideline on caring for children with autism in the acute setting.

If patient satisfaction with a clinical guideline is evaluated, it is important that there is clarity over what is being assessed. The general tendency to be grateful to healthcare professionals may obscure the evaluation of a clinical guideline, or general complaints may override the actual area being explored. Artefactual effects from the overall healthcare experience should therefore be addressed in designing evaluation tools.

Staff perspectives should also be sought in the evaluation of clinical guidelines. This may include whether staff view patient outcomes as being improved, whether they perceive the guideline as improving cost-effectiveness or use of resources, whether a guideline is practical and user-friendly and whether the recommendations are useful and implementable in practice.

The guideline evaluation process needs to clearly feed into the ongoing guideline development process. If part of a guideline is found to be impractical, or the wording unclear or misleading, this needs to be addressed and the guideline amended. If individuals cannot see how their evaluation alters events, they are unlikely to continue to participate in evaluation activities and may feel that their views are not listened to.

As was discussed in Chapter 5, altering clinical guidelines soon after they have been produced and implemented is likely to be costly and may be confusing for staff. This emphasises the value of piloting clinical guidelines prior to their widespread use. However, if staff are required to evaluate guidelines and negative evaluation is not seen to be acted upon, they need to know why this is.

EDITORIAL INDEPENDENCE

AGREE (2001) state that clinical guidelines should be editorially independent and that any conflicts of interest which might have affected their development should be made explicit. Guideline development may be funded locally, for example by a Primary Care Trust, or may have attracted external funding, for example from the DoH, a charity or a pharmaceutical company. The funding of a guideline should not affect the development process or the recommendations made. For example, if a drug company funds the development of a clinical guideline, there should be no influence from them over how the guideline is developed or whether their drugs are recommended for use. However, it introduces a potential for bias, and all funding sources for the guideline should therefore be stated. There may also be potential conflicts of interest for members of the development group. For example, if a member of the development group is undertaking research on the topic covered by the guideline and is funded by a pharmaceutical company (SIGN, 2005). In some circumstances, such individuals should not be involved in guideline development; however, in others their conflict of interest would not preclude them being involved but is something which the development group should be aware of. These issues being made explicit indicate that the group were open about their funding sources and potential biases or conflicts of interest and took appropriate steps to minimise the effects of these. Being open about funding and conflicts of interest also demonstrates confidence that the guideline group feel that these factors were not allowed to bias guideline development, and that they have nothing to hide.

SUMMARY

Using clinical guidelines and care protocols appropriately and to improve patient care includes deciding when not to use them. Not all clinical guidelines or care protocols are of a high standard (Christiaens *et al.*, 2004). A repeated theme in previous chapters has been that being called a clinical guideline or care protocol does not, of itself, give any indication of the quality of a document. Therefore, before a decision is made to use a clinical guideline or care protocol, its quality should be assessed. A part of the decision over whether or not to use a clinical guideline or care protocol is to decide whether it is suitable for a particular practice setting. A clinical guideline may itself be of good quality, but for it to enhance the quality of care it must be used in appropriate situations. Finally, as well as its apparent quality and applicability, the actual effectiveness of clinical guidelines in improving care must also be evaluated.

Although there are a number of indicators of the quality of a clinical guideline, having a framework to assess this means that the evaluation is more likely to be systematic. The AGREE Collaboration have issued guidance which is internationally agreed to be a valid way of assessing the quality of guidelines (AGREE, 2001). The criteria suggested by AGREE include that the guideline should have a clear statement of purpose, have evidence of appropriate stakeholder involvement, have been rigorously developed, be clearly presented, applicable and editorially independent.

Guidelines should be assessed prior to their use. However, they should also be subject to ongoing evaluation to determine if they are used and continue to be used, if they produce and continue to produce benefits in patient care and if they are cost-effective.

7

Implementing Guidance

The transfer of research findings into practice has always presented challenges, even when the advantages outlined in the research are strong (Davies, 2002; Feasey and Fox, 2001). The concept of evidence-based practice and the use of clinical guidelines and care protocols should make the transfer of evidence into practice more straightforward, as their central theme is that the practical implications of the evidence should be made clear. However, Ricart *et al.* (2003) and Thomas *et al.* (2003) identify that the use of evidence in practice often continues to fall short of expectations. Despite a large number of recommendations and guidelines being issued by organisations such as NICE, these are often not used in practice, or delays occur in their implementation (Shannon, 2003; Sheldon *et al.*, 2004). Ryan *et al.* (2004) report no significant change in the use of hip prostheses in the NHS following NICE guidance on this subject being released and Wathen and Dean (2004) found that NICE guidance, of itself, made little impact on GPs' prescriptions.

This may, at least in part, be because, as Berenholtz and Pronovost (2003) identify – although considerable effort is often expended in seeking evidence, evaluating this and describing its practical implications – how it will be put into practice and how guidance will be implemented frequently receives scant attention. This may also apply to clinical guidelines and care protocols. However accurate a reflection of the current best evidence a clinical guideline or care protocol is, and however much it would enhance care, unless it is used in practice, the time taken to develop it will not be well spent and it will be of no real value to patients. If clinical guidelines and care protocols are to enhance care provision, the process and practicalities of implementing them must therefore be given equal consideration to their development.

The time and effort which it can take to achieve changes in practice should not be underestimated. Although the time that it can take for clinical guidelines or care protocols to become standard practice may be considerable, particularly where they require a significant change in practice, every effort should be made to make their implementation as rapid as possible. It is likely that if the timeframe for implementing new evidence is significant the evidence concerning an area of practice will have changed and that the development of new techniques, therapeutic agents or approaches to care provision will mean that what was considered 'best practice' no longer is. The cost of interventions may also change significantly in a five-year period. If guidance takes this long to come into effect, it is therefore likely that it will not produce care based on the current best evidence, and may even encourage out-of-date practice.

This chapter therefore considers some of the factors which must be taken into account when implementing clinical guidelines and care protocols. Notwithstanding the recommendations in this chapter, the assumption should not be made that because a guideline or protocol exists, even one which has been developed by a national body such as SIGN or NICE, it must be used. As Chapter 6 identified, not all guidelines or protocols are of good quality, and before expending effort in effecting changes in practice whether or not these changes are derived from sound guidance must be established. This chapter refers to implementing guidance that has been evaluated and found to be based on sound evidence.

CLEAR AND AVAILABLE INFORMATION

We have probably all experienced the irritation of great advice after the event. My first car was a Renault 5. Renault 5s are, it turns out, notorious for taking a bit of encouragement to start, especially in the winter. Mine was no exception. It coughed and spluttered, covered the road in the kind of cloud of smoke more usually associated with a war zone, woke everyone within ten miles and eventually fired, only to cut out again in the middle of the first big junction or roundabout of the day. Far from being the sedentary way to travel, driving my car through busy junctions on a cold morning was adrenaline sport. Nothing that a PICU could throw my way even began to compete with the challenge of starting the car and getting from Brighton to London for an early shift in winter. Once my Renault 5 experience had begun, everyone else began sharing with me their 'starting a Renault 5' horror stories. It was the kind of information I would have preferred to have received before buying the car.

It has been suggested that one reason why research is not used in practice is that staff are often unaware of its existence (Feasey and Fox, 2001). One of the intentions of clinical guidelines and care protocols is to overcome this problem by making clear what evidence is available and how this applies to practice. However, staff must still be aware of the existence of clinical guidelines or care protocols in order to be able to use them. To avoid this problem, how clinical guidelines or care protocols will be brought to the attention of frontline staff merits attention. It will be of little value for a Trust's chief executive to know that new guidance exists regarding the best way to manage seizures in the accident and emergency department if this is not known by the staff in the department itself. It is of greater value for the clinical director of A & E to know this than the chief executive, but it is of greatest value for all the staff in the accident and emergency department, who will be providing immediate treatment to patients, to know this. Effective methods of disseminating guidance to appropriate audiences is a vital part of making clinical guidelines and care protocols a reality in practice.

Where national guidance is issued by organisations such as NICE or SIGN, how this will be distilled into practice areas and to individual staff is an essential consideration if practice is to change. National guidelines are posted on the NICE and SIGN websites and are also disseminated to individuals who have expressed an interest or are on the organisations' mailing lists, and to NHS Trusts and throughout the NHS in Scotland. However, such distribution does not guarantee that the guidance is seen by the staff who will actually be providing care. Mechanisms by which new national guidance will be cascaded to frontline staff must therefore be devised. The distribution of SIGN guidelines in Scotland is organised within each NHS board by local distribution coordinators, who are often also responsible for facilitating the implementation of the guidance that they distribute. In the case of locally developed guidelines, how all staff within a Trust, clinical area or directorate will be made aware of new clinical guidelines or care protocols also requires consideration. It may be tempting to think that because guidance is developed locally all staff will be aware of its existence. However, it is possible, even when guidance is developed at ward level, for some staff to be unaware of its existence, even after it has supposedly been implemented. The same principle applies to guidance which is being adopted from other organisations, for example guidance from the National Electronic Library for Health's bank of protocols.

Knowing that guidance is available is the start point for using clinical guidelines or care protocols. However, for them to actually be used, staff must be able to access them with relative ease. One of the most commonly cited reasons for evidence-based practice not being achieved is a lack of time (Lawrie *et al.*, 2000; Frost *et al.*, 2003; Thomas *et al.*, 2003; Bhandari *et al.*, 2003). Staff are therefore more likely to use clinical guidelines and care protocols if they can find and use them with minimum inconvenience and without an unnecessary increase in their workload. Unless they perceive their need for guidance to be very strong, awareness that a guideline may exist somewhere is unlikely to prompt staff to find and use this when other competing priorities exist. For instance, a GP who has managed children with eczema for many years with what seems to be relatively good results may not be prepared to spend considerable time and effort finding and deciphering a new guideline on the subject in the middle of a busy schedule of appointments. However, if a clear and concise guideline is easily accessible in his surgery, he may be more inclined to use it. Guidelines should, therefore, be easily physically accessible to practitioners in the clinical setting (Lawrie *et al.*, 2000; Scott *et al.*, 2000).

Making guidance accessible includes considering whether any electronic media required to access it is available to practitioners and whether practitioners are conversant with its use. For example, interactive electronic guidelines may appear very useful but, unless the hardware which staff have access to is of sufficient quantity and quality to allow the rapid access to and downloading of information the guidance might not be easily accessible. Given the competing demands on their time, if staff must search for a free computer and then having achieved this, find that the access to guideline pages is slow, they may well decide to initiate the treatment or care which they usually give rather than waiting for the up-to-date information to appear. Equally, if the hardware needed is not close to patient-care areas, it is less likely that staff will access and use it. If a nurse is caring for a group of highly dependent patients on a general medical ward, it is unlikely that they will have time to go and sit in the office to seek out the electronic version of the RCN's guideline on pressure-relieving devices to decide what to use for a newly admitted patient. It is much more likely that they will go to the ward cupboard and see what is available, and, based on their existing knowledge and accepted practice, select a device. If a computer terminal is available in the high-dependency bay in which the patients are cared for, it is slightly more likely that electronic guidelines will be used.

The assumption should not be made that all staff are conversant with using electronic media, and a busy shift is not a time when learning information-technology skills will be a high priority. (On children's wards, this problem can usually be overcome by asking a child under the age of five to assist.) However, this kind of support cannot be guaranteed, and, if electronic guidelines are to be used, attention needs to be given to the location and quality of equipment and to whether all staff are conversant with its use.

Once staff are aware of and can access guidance, the way in which this is presented needs to be clear and user-friendly (McKinlay, 2004). A busy clinician will not want to spend a large amount of time working out what a guideline says and what this means. If guidelines are intended to enable practitioners to provide care confidently, knowing that they have taken what is thought to be the right course of action, the guidance given needs to facilitate this. The wording of guidelines should be specific, unambiguous, concise and, as far as possible, concrete, with definite statements about what should be done and when (Michie and Johnston, 2004). Although there are likely to be a variety of options in many situations, what should be done in each case should be clear. For example, if there is an instruction to check a patient's blood pressure postoperatively, what action should be taken if this is normal, high or low should be clear.

Guideline statements should therefore be clear and logical. As well as improving the use of clinical guidelines and care protocols, having clear and unequivocal guidance will make it easier to determine if a guideline has been followed. This should in turn assist with the process of guideline evaluation.

As well as individual guidelines being clear, there should be clarity for practitioners over what guidance should be followed. If more than one set of guidelines exist, for example local and national guidelines, staff should know which set of instructions they are expected to adhere to (Morris, 2001). One of the remits of NICE and SIGN is to provide clear national guidance, and thus to some extent to overcome this problem, but there are cases where national guidance has been adapted to suit local circumstances, or where the guidance issued by NICE and other specialist organisations differs. For example, the guidelines issued by the British Hypertension Society and NICE differ in some respects (Poulter, 2004) and practitioners need clarity over which set of advice to follow. Where local guidance is being used, there may be differences in the guidance given, for example, between Primary Care Trusts and Acute Trusts, which may be confusing when patients with chronic conditions who are usually cared for at home are admitted to hospital. There may be good reasons for variations in guidance between community and hospital, for example related to equipment used or the different environment in which procedures are being carried out, but what guidance should be followed, when and why should be clear to all parties.

REASONS FOR USING GUIDELINES

Staff need to be convinced that the reasons for any change in practice demanded by new guidelines are sufficient to merit them investing their time. Staff may choose to ignore guidelines because they are not persuaded that the evidence which has informed their development is of high quality, or of their relevance to the setting in which they are proposed, or because they see no problem with current practice and therefore no reason to alter it (Flottorp and Oxman, 2003; Ricart *et al.*, 2003; Tracy *et al.*, 2003). How staff can be involved in guideline development is discussed later in this chapter; however, where guidance that has been developed by third parties is introduced, its implementation is most likely to be successful if local opinion leaders, or colleagues who are seen as trustworthy or credible in practice rather than detached national bodies, are seen to promote its use (National Health and Medical Research Council, 2000). Individuals who are respected by staff and thought to understand the pressures which they face are more likely to have credibility with those who will be using guidelines than unknown government agencies or professional organisations. Their endorsement of guidance is therefore likely to be more meaningful to frontline staff than the fact that an organisation such as NICE or SIGN have issued it. Such individuals can also evaluate the information contained in national guidelines, determine how this fits the local context and thus assist staff to see how national guidance can be implemented locally and why this is worthwhile. This may mean that, while the guidance issued by national bodies is not followed to the word, the principles which

Clinical Guidelines and Care Protocols

it contains are adhered to, rather than guidance being discarded as irrelevant or being implemented in name but not in reality.

Although local opinion leaders are cited as being important in guideline implementation, exactly who will be appropriate for this role requires some thought. It will not usually be possible for national organisations, such as SIGN or NICE, to determine who, in individual organisations, is the best person to cascade information to individual staff. National guidance is most likely to be imparted to managers in the first instance, with the expectation that they will make decisions regarding how this should be shared. In some cases, managers are those best placed to give information to and influence their staff, but this is not always so. Frontline staff may not always be convinced that their managers understand the practical implications of guidance or the pressures that they work under.

One responsibility of managers is therefore to identify the individuals best placed to impart information about national guidance to direct caregivers. There is no easy answer to who this should be, and one aspect of management expertise is to be aware of the dynamics of teams within organisations and to use this to determine who staff will trust in individual cases. Having specialist staff available to provide input and support and to discuss with groups of staff the practicalities of the recommendations which have been made may be useful (Frost *et al.*, 2003). Although specialist staff can be invaluable for providing information, explaining guidance and the rationale for this, general staff still need to be convinced that staff from specialist centres or units understand the implications which guidance has for them and the area that they work in.

The ideal would be to involve specialist staff alongside local facilitators, such as respected colleagues, so that the specialist knowledge can be understood and used but guidance also adapted to local circumstances or realities in such a way that implementation will be accepted as being possible and appropriate. However, the grade or job specification of those who are respected and will be listened to locally cannot be predetermined.

Using new guidelines is likely to involve a degree of change of practice, which will require them to make some additional effort over and above that which they normally make. Compliance is therefore more likely if the benefits of the effort which they are required to make are known. Clinical guidelines should be based on the best evidence of clinical efficacy and cost-effectiveness, and the benefits in clinical or cost terms may therefore be able to be shared with staff to encourage guideline use. There may also already be results from the implementation of guidance in other areas which can be used to demonstrate that benefits have been seen in real-world practice rather than in terms of theoretical risk:benefit calculations.

As Chapter 6 identified, the design of clinical guidelines and care protocols should include mechanisms for feedback on the benefits and costs of any change in practice. A process whereby guideline use can be evaluated should therefore be in place when new guidance is implemented, and staff should be aware of how and when the evaluation data will be available. It is likely to be helpful for staff to know what benefits to them and their patients are expected from guideline use, and how and when they will know whether these are achieved at the outset. If it is known that the results of implementing a new protocol will take a year to show benefit, this should be made clear so that staff do not feel that no feedback is forthcoming. If the benefits of following a new set of guidance are borderline for staff or patients, the effort involved in instigating, implementing and maintaining change is unlikely to be a priority within the competing claims on staff time. There is also an argument that, if benefits are indeed borderline, guideline implementation should not be attempted if the time and effort required for it is not a good use of resources.

Including clinical guidelines in quality-improvement processes and audit cycles can be useful in demonstrating the effect which they have on practice. It is also useful to link evaluation of new practice to audit so that there is coherence between the many quality-related tasks, which staff are obliged to engage in, in order that staff can see the relevance of audit to practice, and also to reduce any replication of evaluative work. However, as Chapters 6 and 11 discuss, using guidelines as a part of quality-control mechanisms may be both beneficial and problematic. There is a potential for guideline use rather than quality of care to become the focus. Nevertheless, if audit processes are designed so as to include a method of demonstrating whether or not following clinical guidelines or care protocols contributes to quality of care, not just whether they are used, they may be useful in this respect.

USER INVOLVEMENT

Whether staff have positive or negative attitudes towards a new approach to practice is a major factor affecting its implementation. A vital element of successfully implementing clinical guidelines or care protocols will therefore be to create positive attitudes in staff towards their use.

Deshpande *et al.* (2003) identify that healthcare staff can see the imposition of guidance as a threat to their professional autonomy. This can make them reluctant to accept and use them even if they are of good quality. User involvement in guideline development and in decisions regarding their use may reduce this problem. However, although the involvement of staff is almost universally cited as an important part of change management, the use of clinical guidelines and care protocols may not be truly optional, as local or national guidance may be centrally developed and, as subsequent chapters will discuss, to a degree, imposed on staff. Individual practitioners are always expected to decide whether any guidance is appropriate in individual cases. The overall expectation is that guidance issued by organisations such as NICE and SIGN will be adhered to, although there is evidence that this is not the case (Ryan *et al.*, 2004; Wathen and Dean, 2004; Shannon, 2003; Sheldon *et al.*,

2004). The implications of this for professional freedom are discussed in more detail in Chapter 8. However, consideration must be given to how the greatest possible degree of user ownership and autonomy should be facilitated with national guidance if its use is to be increased.

One step towards achieving greater use of national guidance is to determine how the priorities of guideline developers and staff who are expected to implement these can be matched. Although national guidelines are intended to enhance the clinical efficacy and cost-effectiveness of care, national agendas and local priorities will not always match (Brooks and Barrett, 2003). In addition, the priorities of managers and frontline clinical staff may not be the same. The pressures upon central organisations such as NICE, Trust managers and staff providing direct care are also likely to differ. However, it is generally frontline staff who provide direct care whose cooperation is essential for the recommendations in clinical guidelines or care protocols to become a reality for those receiving care.

Given the competing claims on staff time, if an issue is not seen as problematic or especially important by practitioners, changing practice is unlikely to be a priority (Semin-Goossens *et al.*, 2003). This will be the case even when it may be identified as a national priority. For example, the prevention of heart disease is a national priority, and most healthcare staff would agree that this is, in principle, a good thing. However, implementing a new guideline on this may not be the day-to-day priority of staff on a cardiac unit who have acute stabilisation of patients following myocardial infarction, rehabilitation of patients with cardiac disease or injury and health-promotion activities to undertake, especially if there are already health-promotion processes in place which seem to work reasonably well.

Thus, for the use of national clinical guidelines and care protocols to become a reality, identification of local priorities (including the priorities of local NHS or Primary Care Trusts and individual wards or caseloads), how these may interface with national priorities and how the priorities of managers and clinical staff can be reconciled is important. How, for example, the requirement for managers to demonstrate that central targets have been met can be achieved alongside the range of direct care demands placed on frontline staff may need to be unravelled. This will include discussions on how the competing priorities of government, clinical staff and Trust or unit managers can be addressed in which individuals and staff groups genuinely seek to understand the perspectives of others. Where a directorate is required to produce a care protocol on how coronary heart disease will be prevented, the development and documentation of a formal protocol may be seen by clinical staff as less important than actually providing the input on heart-disease prevention to patients, which they always do regardless of a documented protocol. It may also be that staff on a cardiac unit feel that teaching staff about providing care to those immediately post myocardial infarction in order to achieve acute stability is a greater priority than teaching staff about a health-promotion protocol for patients on discharge. However, from a managerial perspective, significant financial losses may result from the non-production or nonimplementation of a protocol. This may have staffing implications and may therefore impact on direct patient care. Open discussion in such situations may enable compromises to be reached or additional support to be made available for the development or implementation of required guidelines or protocols. Other moves which may enhance local ownership include local staff deciding exactly how they will implement an imposed guideline, what aspects of it they will adopt wholesale and what needs adaptation, what interim targets they will set and how adopting national guidelines may also enable local priorities to be addressed.

This may require considerable time and effort, and in some cases a change in a culture in which central agencies such as NICE, managers and staff are seen as separate entities. This is not easy to achieve, and changing organisational culture is not the work of an afternoon. However, it may in many cases be essential if clinical guidelines and care protocols which are imposed on organisations or individual areas of practice are to be implemented successfully.

User involvement includes all levels of staff and all staff who are affected by the aspect of care in question, and interdisciplinary collaboration as well as collaboration between grades of staff, managers and frontline staff is also usually necessary (National Health and Medical Research Council, 2000; Lewis and Orland, 2004). For example, junior doctors agreeing with their consultants that they will adhere to set protocols relating to preoperative fasting will not guarantee overall compliance if the nurses on surgical wards are unwilling to follow these protocols. As well as the staff who will provide hands-on care, cooperation includes those who may feel they have a vested interest in the guidance given, those whose goodwill will be necessary for the smooth running of any transition period and those who may be involved in the funding needed for any change to occur.

These interpersonal, interdisciplinary and intradisciplinary aspects of guideline implementation and the matching of local and national priorities may be the most complex, and time-consuming, factors involved, but they are also the aspects which can most affect guideline use. It is possible that, where national targets and aims do not match local priorities but there is significant pressure to produce results, a tokenistic approach to guideline implementation will occur, in which it appears that guidelines are used, when in reality they are available but not actually implemented. This includes individual clinical staff claiming to adhere to guidance when in fact they do not, or entire Trusts claiming to have adopted guidance when they have not. There is little doubt that the political expediency of massaging results to make it appear that targets are met has superseded absolute honesty in a number of cases (Smith, 2003). This may be politically and financially expedient; however, if clinical guidelines and care protocols are to be meaningfully used, and their value in relation to patient care really evaluated, then how their actual use, rather than their acceptance in name only, can be facilitated merits considerable effort. Quality-control mechanisms in healthcare are often described as a paper exercise, and a requirement to tick the right boxes, which has little relevance to patient care. This may well be so; however, if it is to change, staff at all levels must be willing to engage in real debate over why certain quality mechanisms, guidelines or protocols are or are not used or useful.

Junior or frontline staff are generally those who are ultimately required to implement new practice and whose cooperation is therefore crucial to the success of innovations. For this reason, the bottom-up approach to implementing change is often advocated (Gough, 2001). This ideally means that frontline staff identify a practice issue which needs to be addressed, and that from this the process by which changes in practice emerge is commenced, with these therefore being perceived as relevant by frontline staff. It also means that from the outset and at every point those who will be using new practice are involved and in fact lead change. In some cases, clinical guidelines or care protocols will be developed as a direct result of an identified need, and this model can be followed. However, in the case of national guidelines, or guidelines which are dictated by national agendas, guidance will, in many respects, be imposed. In these situations, managers may be required to find ways in which they can encourage staff to use imposed guidance or to explore ways in which this can be harnessed to local need. Here, involving frontline staff and ascertaining their views on how guidance can be made locally relevant, as detailed above, may be the closest that can be achieved to the ideal bottom-up approach to change management.

Although the bottom-up approach to change management is usually advocated, Gollop (2003) and Wyatt *et al.* (1998) identify that, while the initiation of change by frontline staff is a valuable approach, junior staff require support from senior colleagues to effect change. Feasey and Fox (2001) identify that nurses do not always feel they have the authority to change patient care or that the organisations within which they work will allow them to implement changes in practice even when they see this as important. Junior medical staff have cited senior colleagues and their institutions as preventing them from implementing evidence-based recommendations (Bhandari *et al.*, 2003). Thus, although initiation of change by junior or frontline staff may appear attractive, change management, and in this case the introduction of clinical guidelines or care protocols, also requires involvement of and support from all levels of staff (Feasey and Fox, 2001). Although it may seem that senior staff are more likely to accept national clinical guidelines or care protocols, because of greater awareness of policy issues, this may not be the case. Senior clinical staff may be less willing to change practice which has been established over years than junior staff. It is also possible that senior staff may be more appropriately resistant to change or demand knowledge on the quality of the evidence presented and have a greater influence to refute change on the basis of unconvincing evidence. Resistance to change is not necessarily negative; questioning of imposed or suggested change is an essential part of ensuring that the proposed new practice is appropriate. Involving senior staff is therefore as important as gaining the support of junior staff and will assist in making sure that the right questions have been asked and that the necessary support for junior staff is available.

Although user involvement is often cited as a major facilitator of change management, user involvement does not guarantee compliance. Livesey (2005) cites a multiagency protocol regarding sudden childhood death as being poorly implemented despite being drawn up in collaboration with the relevant disciplines and approved by coroners, area child protection committees and senior managers. The suggestion from this work is that as well as user involvement strong lines of accountability for guideline implementation are needed and that statutory backing may also be necessary. Thus, as well as all levels of staff being involved in guideline implementation locally, it may be that sanction and even dictates from statutory bodies are needed for guideline implementation to work, and that this should be initial and ongoing. It is therefore clear that, although it is often tempting to discuss change management as a simple process whereby involving frontline staff will facilitate change, the reality is that all levels of staff need to be simultaneously involved and that, although imposed national guidance presents challenges, the backing of national bodies may be needed to enable staff to effect change. Redfern and Christian (2003) state that the management of change in healthcare is often more likely to take a dynamic, disorderly and uncertain route than a rational, linear one because of the complexities of the organisation. The same is true for who should be involved, and in what sequence, and a simple model of change management may be inadequate in many cases.

Regardless of the precise approach used, for change to occur strong leadership is needed (Buonocore, 2004; Livesey, 2005). This does not mean that senior personnel must manage the change process, but, given the complexity of the introduction of new guidance, strong overall coordination and management of the change in question is needed. In change processes, there is a need for considerable work to plan the implementation of new approaches, followed by their actual implementation and then for new processes to sustain any changes in practice and evaluate the new practice. This will be helped by having staff who are able to dedicate time to coordinating and monitoring these processes. In addition, if strong leadership does not exist, it is unlikely that change will be effected or sustained. There are likely to be some interested parties who immediately embrace new practice, a number who will never willingly change their practice and a large proportion who, all things being equal, will comply, but for whom this is not a priority. Encouraging this last group to be involved, and sustaining their motivation and that of the enthusiastic group, while also encouraging participation from those who would prefer to abstain, is a task which requires sustained effort and effective leadership.

Leadership may need to be by different individuals and at different levels, for example Trust level, ward level and profession level.

RESOURCES

Ricart *et al.* (2003) identify a lack of resources, amongst which are financial resources, as major factors in cases where there is a failure to implement evidence-based recommendations or guidelines. Financial considerations include the cost of guideline implementation, the necessary equipment, production of guideline statements, the production of summaries for use in everyday practice and staff education. How the cost of implementing new practice interfaces with other priorities, particularly where there is an initial outlay cost from which benefits are ultimately expected but which will not be evident in the short term, is also a consideration. This is especially problematic where the achievement of short-term financial targets, such as yearly budgets, is the measured outcome. This means that, where they are to be implemented, the planning and evaluation of new guidelines should include a realistic range of evaluative tools which reflect the timing of benefit and any initial expected mismatch in cost and benefit analysis, such as delayed financial benefit despite initial set-up costs. It also demonstrates why managerial support as well as support from frontline staff is needed and why decisions about adopting guidelines must include how manageable this is for the organisation in question at any given point in time.

Nonetheless, the cost in financial terms arising from any failure to meet targets which are locally or nationally set, the cost should legal action be taken against an NHS Trust where available evidence is not used and the personal cost to staff who may be accused of malpractice in such situations must also be taken into account. This is likely to be one area in which managers and frontline staff can usefully engage in discussions, as their viewpoints may not match. It is also a reason why, although many healthcare staff may find awareness of or involvement in political and managerial issues an unwelcome detractor from direct care activities, they should be aware of the implications of non-adherence to national targets and standards. This includes how financial penalties may ultimately impact upon direct care and even their own ongoing employment.

LOW PRIORITY

Time may be a major issue in implementing new guidance. Healthcare professionals have multiple and competing demands on their time and resources, one of which is the time required to effect the implementation of new guidance at any given time. This includes the time taken for education and training in guideline use, but also the effort required to seek and follow new guidance on a day-to-day basis rather than carrying out care as usual.

It is often suggested that evidence-based practice fails because it is seen as having lower priority than the other competing demands on healthcare professionals' time (Frost *et al.*, 2003; Lawrie *et al.*, 2000; Thomas *et al.*, 2003; Bhandari *et al.*, 2003). Long (2003) has identified that quality improvement is often considered by clinicians to be yet another task to be added to their already heavy workloads. Even where the relative advantages of guideline use are high, the time taken to implement them or to find and use them on a day-to-day basis may seem overwhelming and unmerited in comparison to other demands. There are many reasons why using evidence to inform practice may be low priority, and, as identified by Shannon (2003), in some cases the necessary precursors to implementing new protocols or guidelines in terms of diagnostic processes or infrastructure may take some time to set up and achieve even where there is great enthusiasm for this. For example, the guidelines on the management of multiple sclerosis are said to require a tripling of the number of neurologists and the number of nurse specialists to be doubled (Jain, 2003). This is a task which, it can be assumed, cannot be achieved in a short timeframe if quality as well as quantity of staff is the aim. Delays in guideline implementation because of this type of practical issue are inevitable. Nonetheless, where quality guidelines exist but are not implemented because this is seen as a low priority the reason for this must be explored.

The effectiveness of direct patient care is central to the quality of healthcare (Thompson, 2000). The NMC (2002) make clear that providing high-quality care based on the current best evidence is the responsibility of nurses, and the GMC (2005) also suggest that medical staff should provide what they believe to be the best available care. Therefore, where using what is considered to be the best, most up-to-date evidence to inform practice appears to have become low priority, why this is the case must be explored and questions asked about the individual or organisation's priorities. Professionally and legally, where care protocols or clinical guidelines are not followed, staff must be able to justify why this is the case. Although determining priorities in any given situation is the responsibility of each practitioner, and there will be times when disregarding a guideline or protocol is entirely appropriate, the ethos of being busy providing care which is of unproven value must be questioned. The risk is that individuals are busy providing care which is of no proven value, is of poor quality or is even dangerous. Being busy harming patients is not defensible.

PATIENT EXPECTATIONS

Although the focus of implementing clinical guidelines and care protocols is often on staff, patients' responses to new approaches to treatment or care and their expectations should not be underestimated in the equation (Flottorp and Oxman, 2003; Tracy *et al.*, 2003; Ricart *et al.*, 2003). If patients refuse to accept care as outlined in clinical guidelines and care protocols, except in very specific circumstances, these cannot be adhered to however much staff may wish to use the guidance in question. As well as effort being expended in assisting staff to embrace guidelines and protocols, attention must therefore be given to patient acceptance of these and how this can be facilitated. In the same way that there is little point in spending a great deal of time developing guidelines which staff will not use, there is little point in expending significant effort in developing guidance and educating staff on its use if the recipients of care do not accept it.

Patient choice, as will be discussed in Chapter 9, is an important part of healthcare, and a culture of paternalism is no longer seen as acceptable. Coercion by any means to follow guidance is therefore not acceptable. Making patients aware of the benefits, as well as risks or disadvantages, of recommended treatment or care to assist them to make an informed choice is the aim. The balance between an informed choice and coercion may be difficult to achieve, and there may be strong pressure to persuade patients to comply with recommendations which assist Trusts to meet national targets. Individual practitioners may also find it hard not to impose their own beliefs and values on patients and thus encourage them towards a route which may not be that individual's choice. Informed decision-making is the aim in healthcare, and enthusiasm by staff for what they see as best, to follow guidance or achieve targets does not justify coercion. There may, nonetheless, be instances where guidelines are unattractive to patients because they have not been given adequate information, or because of practical problems or concerns which are nothing to do with the medical, technical or care input per se. In these cases, practical aspects of care can be managed so that objections are overcome or assistance given, for example timing of treatment or location. Whether patients do not wish to accept a certain approach to care because they do not want the treatment itself, or do not want the associated practical problems or see these as insurmountable, should be made clear. If appropriate and possible, mechanisms can then be put into place to make recommended courses of action more acceptable to them.

Practitioners must therefore distinguish between attempting to coerce patients because of any possible financial implications for Trusts for the non-achievement of targets, personal beliefs or professional agendas and giving patients sufficient information to achieve a truly informed choice.

SUMMARY

The way in which clinical guidelines or care protocols will be implemented merits as much attention as the process of developing the documents which provide guidance. Although this stage often receives less attention, without it the work involved in developing clinical guidelines and care protocols may be wasted and patient care remain unaffected.

For guidelines to be appropriately used, practitioners must be aware of their existence and be able to access these, and they must be presented in a clear, user-friendly format (Lawrie *et al.*, 2000; Scott *et al.*, 2000). How all staff can be made aware of the existence of new guidance merits attention, and how this can be achieved in a manner which encourages compliance is an even greater challenge. As anyone who has sat in the 'quiet coach' on a train, where mobile phones are absolutely forbidden, knows, there are those who know about and follow the guidance/rules, those who are genuinely unaware of guidance/rules, those who are aware but pretend they are not and act innocently when confronted and those who know and yet ignore the guidance/rules and are pleased to be seen doing so. If guidelines are to be more successful than mobile-phone rules, this requires some attention. When the dissemination and implementation of evidence in practice is planned, strategies to involve all levels of staff and all disciplines involved should be included. Evaluation strategies should accompany guideline implementation, and feedback mechanisms should be put in place so that staff can determine whether the time and effort which they are expending in adopting new guidance is worthwhile. Despite initiatives which are seen as local priorities or relevant by users usually being more successful, clinical guideline use is likely to be influenced by political and economic considerations. Therefore, open discussion between all staff is needed so that the needs and priorities of each and how actions and decisions taken by each impact on the others can be understood and common aims reached.

In the planning and implementation of guideline use, the likelihood of this guidance being acceptable to patients should not be overlooked. Although patient autonomy and choice remain key to all healthcare, where a lack of information or practicalities prevent guidelines being acceptable to patients, how these problems can be overcome should be considered.

Evidence-based practice is not achieved by the unthinking implementation of guidelines or recommendations (Hewitt-Taylor, 2003). However, where guidance is not implemented in practice because this is seen as low priority, despite it outlining the best course of action in a given situation, the reason for this must be clear. Time factors are an important consideration, but, where there is a perception that providing high-quality care is not a priority, practitioners should be aware that the rationale for this must be identifiable and justifiable in legal and professional terms.

8

Expertise and Autonomy

Evidence-based practice as described by Sackett *et al.* (1996) and Di Censo *et al.* (1998) emphasises the centrality of healthcare staff using their expert judgement to decide when and how evidence should be used in practice. Clinical guidelines from NICE also come with the caveat that practitioners should exercise their clinical judgement over whether or not to use them in each unique patient circumstance (NICE, 2005b). Professional expertise should therefore be a central part of the use of clinical guidelines and care protocols. This includes expert opinion feeding into the development of guidance as described in Chapter 5, and the individual clinical expertise that should direct the appropriate application of guidance to everyday practice.

However, a criticism which is often levelled at the concept of evidence-based practice in general, and the use of clinical guidelines and care protocols in particular, is that it devalues clinical expertise and reduces care to a series of prescribed steps which anyone can follow, and which staff are required to follow. Some of the concepts associated with clinical guidelines and care protocols, such as the aim for standardisation of practice (DoH, 2000) and their inclusion in quality-monitoring mechanisms do indeed seem to be at odds with the idea of them being used in conjunction with expert decision-making. The concerns over the devaluing of expertise by a focus on the use of guidelines and protocols include an erosion of the expertise of existing staff and new staff being trained in a manner which encourages them to follow guidelines or protocols rather than being educated in a manner which promotes critical thinking and decision-making. There is also potential for clinical guidelines or care protocols to become the focus of care, rather than seeing care provision as a holistic encounter in which clinical guidelines and care protocols play a part. In addition, developments in healthcare provision may be impeded by an overdependence on inflexible guidelines which dictate what must be done, as there is a risk that nothing outside this will be attempted (Loss and Nagel, 2005).

As well as potentially detracting from professional expertise and the development thereof, healthcare professionals may view clinical guidelines and care protocols as impinging on their professional freedom (Wall *et al.*, 2001; Hughes, 2002). Chapter 11 will discuss the issues of power between professions and government, but for individual professionals the presence of a vast range of clinical guidelines and care protocols may be seen as impairing their ability to act in the manner that they feel is most appropriate in each situation. There is an associated concern that those who decide that in specific cases it would be expedient not to follow an existing care protocol or clinical guideline may be found culpable professionally or in law.

This chapter will therefore, firstly, consider how far clinical guidelines or care protocols impinge on professional autonomy and accountability. It will then consider how guidelines or protocols fit or conflict with the concept of expertise in practice.

PRACTITIONER AUTONOMY AND ACCOUNTABILITY

All registered healthcare staff are accountable for their practice. They have a duty of care to their patients and can be found to be in breach of this duty by their actions or omissions. This accountability includes direct accountability to individual patients, wider accountability to society as a whole because of the trust which is placed in them as professionals and accountability to their profession. They are therefore able to be held to account by law and by their professional body, such as the GMC or NMC. A nurse who administers drugs via an arterial, rather than venous, cannula with resultant damage to the patient is accountable to that individual, to society as a whole because it entrusts them with drug administration and to the profession that they represent and membership of which allows them to administer drugs.

Healthcare professionals' accountability to individuals and society as a whole means that where they are felt to have failed to meet the standards required of them they can be held to account by the law of the country in which they practise. Legal action may be taken against healthcare staff in civil cases, such as where they are accused of negligence. In England, this is covered by the law of tort in which a duty of care was owed to the client and such a duty was not met, with resultant damage to the plaintiff (Fletcher and Buka, 1999). Healthcare professionals may also be accused under criminal law in relation to their practice, for example for murder. The relationship between a healthcare professional and a patient is based on trust, and the law expects more of a professional than it would of non-professionals, because of their privileged position in relation to the trust placed in them by a patient (Fletcher and Buka, 1999).

Healthcare professions such as nursing and medicine have regulatory bodies that oversee practice and have the power of admitting or barring individuals from registration. Professions with this type of self-regulation tend to be allowed the greatest independence and autonomy as there is an expectation that their members will function within accepted parameters and, should they fail to do so, will be subject to professional disciplinary action (Wilmot, 2003). Individuals who practise within such professions can be accused of professional misconduct, which may place their continued registration and thus membership of the profession in jeopardy. This may be associated with a case which is brought against them in law, or may not be. Where a professional is accused both in law and by their governing body, the two decisions on their case, in law and by a professional body, may not always be the same. Although the legal case will be judged by the standards of the profession in question and whether a reasonable professional would have acted in this manner (Fletcher and Buka, 1999), the law and professional standards are different. The decisions reached may, therefore, be different. For example, a physician who is accused of manslaughter may be found innocent of this charge, as it may not be proven that his or her actions or omissions resulted in the death of a patient. The patient may have had multiple pathologies which mean that their actual action cannot be said to have caused death. However, the treatment which they provided may still be seen to fall short of expected professional standards and the trust which the public place in them, and thus they may still be found guilty of professional misconduct. There are therefore two elements to a professional's accountability: their accountability to their profession and their accountability to the individual patient and by extension to society, for acting in the patient's best interests.

Healthcare professionals may also be found to be in breach of their contract of employment if they have acted outside this. They may therefore have legal action taken against them by their employer as well as by an individual patient if they are thought to have acted negligently and to have concurrently been in breach of the agreement between themselves and their employer (Fletcher and Buka, 1999).

As healthcare professionals have this level of accountability, they can also logically expect to have a degree of autonomy or freedom to make decisions. One cannot be held responsible for one's actions if one has no control over them. If practitioners are obliged, absolutely, to follow a course of action, this cannot then be something for which they can be held accountable. If a physician is obliged, absolutely, to prescribe intravenous steroids for all children admitted with an acute asthma attack, they cannot be found guilty of giving inappropriate treatment for doing so. If the physician is allowed to decide, on the basis of the child's history, clinical condition, treatment already given, peak flow recordings and their expertise based on experience, possibly in conjunction with a clinical guideline or care protocol, on what to prescribe, they are accountable for that decision. There are, in fact, few situations in which an individual is absolutely without choice, but many factors exist which decrease choice or ability to decide on a course of action. In the military, 'acting on orders' has been used as a rationale or mitigation for unacceptable behaviour. In other circumstances, the likely reprisals against individuals by other persons or organisations are used in mitigation for crime. However, in healthcare, practitioners expect to enjoy a degree of freedom to make decisions themselves regarding the care of individual patients. Although professions have codes of conduct and ethical principles which guide them, they do not expect, in the same way that military personnel may, to have to 'follow orders'.

There has, nonetheless, been concern that clinical guidelines or care protocols may in effect become orders which must be followed (Loss and Nagel, 2005).This would logically decrease professional accountability, as individuals could safely follow a guidline or protocol, and, regardless of the consequences, remain without blame because they would be seen to be following the orders adopted by their profession and employer. It might even be argued that if they do not follow a care protocol or clinical guideline, they would be guilty of misconduct for not acting in the way that their profession had stated a reasonable healthcare professional should act, and, by not following the rules adopted by their employer, be in breach of contract. One stated intention of care protocols is that they will enable staff to practise with greater safety (NHS Modernisation Agency and NICE, 2004a). However, it seems that staff may be able to practise with greater safety provided they follow prescribed guidelines or protocols, but may be less safe if they fail to do so.

The degree of duress under which professionals are placed to follow guidance is largely dependent upon the guideline or protocol in question and who is obliging them to use it. The consequences of not adhering to guidance also varies. This includes implications for individuals, which may be legal and professional if they fail to follow guidance and there are adverse outcomes or are seen by managers or colleagues as non-compliant or difficult to work with. Failure to have in place or follow guidelines or protocols may also result in financial penalties for orgnisations, for example where targets linked with clinical guidelines or the development of care protocols are not met. If an NHS Trust fails to achieve the implementation of some standards or protocols, they may have reduced ratings awarded to them, with potential financial implications and implications for the degree of self-government which they will be permitted. Where a local Trust has decided not to follow a national guideline, the position for individual practitioners is less clear. For example, the national guidance issued by NICE on induction of labour indicates that, where spontaneous rupture of membranes has occurred, induction of labour should be commenced within 72 hours if spontaneous labour does not ensue. However, if a local guideline suggests a 48-hour wait, a midwife may be taken to task by their employer if they follow national, rather than local, guidelines, although professionally they are acting in what might be seen as a reasonable manner. A great deal will then depend upon the midwife having used appropriate professional judgement and sought informed consent from the woman in question and documented this clearly. Thus, there are no absolutes regarding the consequences of not following guidance, but professionals need to be aware of the possible outcomes.

In all cases, where a patient suffers or claims to have suffered harm, a professional will have to defend their actions, regardless of whether or not they were following clinical guidelines or care protocols. In legal terms, clinical guidelines or care protocols do not obviate the practitioner's responsibility to make appropriate decisions in each individual clinical situation (NICE, 2005b) and do not alter their legal responsibility or duty of care (Hughes, 2002). In UK law, the standards against which a professional will be judged is provided through the input of expert witnesses rather than clinical guidelines. The accepted test of whether or not an individual acted appropriately is still the Bolam Test. This is based on professional opinion of what is acceptable practice and what peers would see as reasonable action. This applies both in civil or criminal court and in professional-conduct hearings. There is little case law pertaining to guideline use, and the existence of a guideline does not make compliance mandatory (Hughes, 2002). However, how the profession as a whole view clinical guidelines or care protocols may affect how those providing expert-witness statements or peer judgement view adherence or otherwise to guidelines. At this point in time, a clinical guideline or care protocol existing is not sufficient rationale for acting or failing to act. It may be a part of the consideration over the appropriateness of an action or omission, but to simply state that a protocol was followed is not defensible in law. Neither will it necessarily be the case that a practitioner is found to be negligent if a guideline or protocol is not followed. SIGN (2005) state that it is unlikely that clinical guidelines will become 'gold standard' statements which can, of themselves, allow conclusions to be reached concerning the appropriateness of a decision. What remains paramount is how the individual practitioner explains and can account for their decision-making in specific cases (Hughes, 2002). However, the move towards an increased use of clinical guidelines and care protocols and the greater number of these covering more aspects of care may create an expectation that these will be used, with the onus more likely to be on a professional to explain why they did not follow a guideline or protocol than why they did so.

Thus, the presence of care protocols or clinical guidelines per se does little to alter a practitioner's legal standing. If they are followed inappropriately, healthcare professionals will still be held accountable for providing care which was not in an individual patient's best interests. If they are not followed where they should be, practitioners will be required to account for why this was. Despite the presence of clinical guidelines or care protocols, healthcare professionals must still exercise their expertise and professional judgement in decision-making.

Notwithstanding this, if the increasing range of care protocols and clinical guidelines means that they become a mainstay of practice, there is a risk that they will erode professional autonomy and decision-making skills. Autonomy is defined as a person's ability to make self-determining choices. Making such choices involves independence and decision-making ability (Lowden, 2002).

Thus, in professional practice, autonomy involves practitioners having the independence to make decisions about the treatment or care which they provide, and the ability to make such decisions. To be autonomous, practitioners will therefore need to have the personal attributes which enable them to function independently, to have the experience of making decisions and to be allowed to make independent decisions. Clinical guidelines and care protocols may impinge on this, if they detract from individuals developing independent decision-making skills and are perceived to dictate what a practitioner must do in a given situation, or at least to provide some degree of duress to follow a prescribed course of action.

Autonomy in practice requires individuals to have the knowledge needed to make decisions and experience in decision-making. In both these areas, there has been concern that using clinical guidelines and care protocols may erode the development and maintenance of autonomy. If clinical guidelines and care protocols become the accepted vehicle for decision-making, knowledge outside of the prescribed steps may be eroded and new practitioners may simply develop knowledge of what is contained in care protocols or clinical guidelines or assume that this is how decisions should always be made. They may also fail to develop familiarity with the process of weighing up the range of factors which influence care and making decisions in individual cases. For existing staff, decision-making skills may become eroded. In the worst-case scenario, this could mean that healthcare professionals enter an era in which they see or can contemplate no alternative to following guidelines or protocols, and lose the essential humanism of care which deals with individuals, not numbers.

The consideration of individuals and their needs, combined with expertise which allows individuals to have the confidence to use common sense rather than obsessively adhering to guidelines or protocols, contributes to humanity in healthcare as well as in other walks of life.

Although practitioners hold professional autonomy dear, it may sometimes be appropriate for decision-making by professionals to be restricted. Healthcare professionals have a duty of care, and the relationship between healthcare staff and patients is based on trust. If an individual professional is found guilty of negligence or other forms of misconduct, one option is that they must undertake a period of supervised practice, in which they are not permitted full autonomy. This is felt to be acceptable as it enhances patient safety and is thus in patients' best interests, and, arguably, those of wider society as the practitioner in question is not to be fully trusted. Autonomy comes hand in hand with responsibility, and practitioners who demonstrate an inability to meet the responsibilities associated with autonomy, through a lack of knowledge, lack of skills or lack of care, may have this restricted. Some would argue that high-profile cases have indicated that NHS Trusts or professional bodies have failed to deal appropriately with practitioners who were not meeting the required standard. This may indicate that the professional groups as a whole have betrayed the public trust in them and thus have not shown themselves to be ready to be allowed full autonomy. One major impetus for the development of national standards was the events in paediatric cardiac surgery at Bristol, following which the public required reassurance that they would be safely cared for by healthcare staff (Kennedy, 2001). Thus, although clinical guidelines and care protocols are not intended to be a punitive strategy, there is, historically, an element in them which is derived from an intention to enforce set standards to protect the public.

However, there is also an argument that in developing a culture in which clinical guidelines and care protocols dictate care, clinical expertise will become eroded or devalued and that over time, despite assurances to the contrary, care will become driven and dictated by care protocols and clinical guidelines. Far from ensuring good standards of care, this may adversely influence the quality of care.

DEFINITION OF EXPERTISE

The Oxford English Dictionary (2001) defines an expert as one who is very knowledgeable about or skilful in a particular area. Expertise in healthcare practice includes knowledge and skills because healthcare staff must appropriately apply knowledge to specific care situations (Sackett *et al.*, 1996; Di Censo *et al.*, 1998). Knowledge alone may make someone an expert if they work in a field where theory is the focus, but, as healthcare involves the application of theory to practice, expertise requires knowledge and skills. For example, a physician may have a very good knowledge of the pathophysiology of septic shock; however, if they cannot recognise a shocked patient, their knowledge does not really contribute to expert practice. A nurse may have good communication skills and be very adept at gaining information from patients, but, unless they have the knowledge to understand the implications of the information which they gather, they are not really able to be described as experts. They may gather information but not act appropriately upon it, for example they may gather information which indicates that a patient is at high risk of suicide, but, unless they can use the information that they have gathered to identify this, their information-gathering skills will not be of great benefit to the patient. There are also individuals who are highly skilled at specific technical tasks, and, although they might be an expert in, for example, setting up a dialysis machine, they would not, on this basis alone, be described as an expert nurse. A surgeon may perform a single procedure correctly, even with great skill; however, if the procedure were unnecessary, or not the correct procedure, or carried out at an inappropriate time, their skill will not detract from the fact that they have not enhanced the patient's health or provided expert care.

Although an individual should possess knowledge and skills to be described as an expert, exactly how healthcare professionals will demonstrate expertise has been the subject of discussion for many years. Woolery (1990) and Benner (1984) suggest that experts can rapidly and accurately assess a situation, make appropriate decisions and instigate care in accordance with these decisions. This ability is developed from a range of knowledge and skills gained from a variety of sources, including their practical knowledge and skills gained from experience, theoretical knowledge, reflection on practice and the refinement of these over time. Benner and Tanner (1987) suggest that experts make decisions by recognising patterns and similarities between the situation that they are presented with and their existing experience, and combine this with common-sense understanding, the skills needed to actually perform care, a sense of salience to recognise and prioritise the most important points in any given situation and deliberative rationality. Elstein and Schwartz (2002) and Diaz (2004) also suggest that experienced physicians frequently use a system of matching cases either to specific previous instances, cases, or to more abstract prototypes.

Although experts are seen as using a bank of experience, knowledge and skills, Meerabeau (1992) suggests that the actual process of expert decision-making is achieved without consciously working through the various alternatives and without conscious awareness of the knowledge which is being used. Experts will almost instantaneously and without conscious thought reach a decision and act upon this. Achieving this kind of rapid, but accurate and multifaceted, decision-making, it is argued, requires intuition (Dreyfus and Dreyfus, 1980; Benner, 1984; Darbyshire, 1994; King and Clark, 2002; James *et al.*, 2003). Indeed, Diaz (2004) identifies that although neurologists use various methods for decision-making, including matching patterns, exhaustive probabilistic and deductive reasoning, errors most often occur because of a lack of intuitive judgement.

The Oxford English Dictionary (2001) defines intuition as 'the ability to understand or know something immediately, without conscious reasoning', while Farrington (1993) describes it as an unanalytical, unstructured, deliberate calculation. This seems to suggest that intuition does not require, or even excludes, reasoning, and contrasts with expertise. However, the intuitive judgement in expert decision-making should not mean that knowledge is lacking but rather that it is so imbedded in the practitioner that they are not consciously aware of using it. This is the almost instantaneous and subconscious reflexive analysis of a variety of factors rather than a conscious step-by-step analysis. From such reflexive, intuitive thinking prompt, high-quality, timely decision-making occurs (Meerabeau, 1992; Higuchi and Donald, 2002). These swift multifaceted deductions of expertise are in contrast to the slower more deliberate thought processes of the novice practitioner. Although they may appear to involve less thought, they in fact involve a much higher quality of thinking.

EXPERIENCE OR EXPERTISE?

Many years of experience do not necessarily create expertise. Some individuals who have been practising for many years provide the rationale for how they provide care as: 'I have always done it this way.' Far from becoming experts, they have become embedded in practice which is based on routines or habits. As Chapter 1 identified, one of the reasons for the move to evidence-based practice has been to get away from care that is based only on it having become accepted practice, not because there is evidence that it is the best method of care provision. Most people have worked with at least one person who has been qualified for many years and is not an expert, and many people have worked with someone who has been qualified for many years and still does not provide a particularly high standard of care. Outside of healthcare, many people have come across individuals who have been driving a car for many years but are not particularly good drivers, and some who are a tad unsafe. Nonetheless, they have never done anything bad enough to lose their licence, and many have never been involved in an accident – possibly because their driving is so bad that everyone keeps a self-preserving distance from them. In the same way in healthcare, some practitioners who are not especially good at their jobs may never have done anything bad enough to be subject to disciplinary action by their employer or professional body. Experience is not, therefore, in healthcare or any other walk of life, any guarantee of expertise.

One way of distinguishing experience and expertise is to identify the level of understanding which has been developed because of experience, and how this has affected an individual's practice, rather than the number of years of practice accrued. King and Clark (2002) and Martin (2002) consider that, for expertise to have developed, individuals must have analysed their experience and used this to refine their practice, not simply accrued years of experience and continued to practise. In a similar way, Paul and Heaslip (1995) suggest that whether or not an individual has engaged in critical reflection helps to distinguish someone who has accrued years of experience and one who has developed expertise. Critical reflection requires an individual to have experience on which to reflect, but to have thought about this experience, its links with other experiences and how it compares with theory on the subject in question to form a bank of information which directs and refines their ongoing practice. This is very different from engagement in ritual care on the basis that 'it has always been done this way' or that this is the prescribed way of practising.

EXPERTISE, CLINICAL GUIDELINES AND CARE PROTOCOLS

The decision-making which experts demonstrate contrasts to following care protocols or clinical guidelines. An expert will arrive at decisions after taking into account all the facets of a situation, albeit rapidly, rather than following a prescribed guideline, a protocol or established practice. The way in which experts make decisions is not linear (Benner, 1984; Rolfe, 1997), and does not necessarily follow clearly defined steps or stages as do care protocols or clinical guidelines. Expert decision-making in healthcare has been likened to the concept of fuzzy logic, which was developed by computer scientists in an attempt to enable computers to mimic expert decision-making (Christiansen and Hewitt-Taylor, in press). Attempts to use logical, analytical formulae that computers could follow to replicate human expertise largely failed because this is not how experts make decisions. Rather than progressing through options and thinking processes in a linear fashion, an expert considers them all at once and attributes each one a different level of importance, depending on the situation. The recognition of this way of reaching decisions led to the development of 'fuzzy logic' (Rolfe, 1997; Kosko, 1994). In fuzzy logic, all the salient parameters of a situation are absorbed rapidly and concurrently weighed up and a decision reached (Rolfe, 1997). While guidelines or protocols tend to be linear, fuzzy logic and expert decision-making both assimilate all the facts, weigh these up and apply them in a sequence which is appropriate in each situation, often in fact applying several at once, for example by observing a patient commencing a new therapy, talking to the patient and thinking ahead to how the data they are gathering from the patient's appearance, speech and vital signs unite to give a picture of how they are responding to therapy and what action should therefore be taken next.

As well as performing all these tasks and assimilating the information from each, an expert will subconsciously decide how much weight each piece of information should carry in the situation in question. A part of the information which is weighed up in expert decision-making will be taking into account clinical guidelines and care protocols, but these will be a part of the decision, not the decision itself. For example, a protocol on administering a new drug may indicate that if the patient's heart rate rises above a certain rate the drug should be stopped. However, in a situation where the patient's normal heart rate is at the higher end of normal pre-drug administration, and they have expressed some concern about the drug, despite consenting to it being administered, and are anxious when it is commenced, a rise in heart rate to just above the stated parameters might lead an expert nurse to decide, dependent on other aspects of the patient's condition and vital signs, to 'wait and see' for a while rather than follow the protocol to stop the drug at once. In this case, the expert has weighed up that the protocol recommends stopping the drug with the fact that the patient did not start from 'normal baseline', which has to be taken into account. In addition, other reasons for a rise in heart rate than the drug, and the effect on the patient's ongoing treatment if a further anxiety is created by stopping the drug so soon, and the fact that if their condition is closely monitored stopping the drug is not an 'emergency', lead to a decision that there is time to 'watch and wait', provided the patient is observed closely.

Benner (1984) suggests that experts do not rigidly follow rules, or see situations as separate parts, but rather take into account a range of sources of information and perceive situations as a whole. Benner (1984), Rolfe (1997), Higuchi and Donald (2002) and Wilkin (2002) also describe experts as providing holistic care rather than proficiently conducting a series of tasks. Benner *et al.* (1992) describe the transition from novice to expert as a movement from reliance on protocols and rules to using abstract principles to direct care, and movement from the perception that a situation is a compilation of relevant parts to seeing the situation as one whole. Thus, while guidelines and protocols have a place in healthcare, they cannot replace, and are indeed in many respects a lower form of practice than, expertise. An expert will not reject guidelines or protocols, but these will be a part, not the entirety, of what informs their decision-making. In addition, as the expert views situations as a whole, not as composite parts, following guidelines or protocols related to one aspect of care will be weighed up by experts in relation to how they pertain to the situation as a whole, not just the element of care to which they directly relate.

Therefore, although experts may, and probably will, use clinical guidelines or care protocols, there is more to practice than this and these will be overridden if other factors indicate that a better way of providing care in a given situation exists. In addition, although the care that experts provide may include following a guideline or protocol, this will be incorporated into the whole picture of care, rather than care being based primarily around the guideline or protocol.

THE SCOPE OF EXPERTISE

In Spain, '*coger*' usually means a form of 'to catch', for example it can be used in reference to taking public transport. In Madrid, if you wish to take a bus, you would be well within your rights to suggest that you would like to '*coger un aútobus.*' A native Spanish speaker (who might therefore be considered an expert in speaking Spanish) found that the same phrase was not so well received in Argentina. In Argentina, '*coger*' is usually used as a vulgar way of expressing sexual activity, and not something that many people would want to engage in with a bus.

Although 'expert practitioners' are referred to, the factors which combine to form expertise in healthcare mean that it is usually situation-specific. Some aspects of the bank of knowledge and experience needed to become an expert will be transferable, but the whole picture view required for holistic, intuitive, expert practice will not be (Higuchi and Donald, 2002). Higuchi and Donald (2002) also suggest that nurses in different specialities use different thinking processes to make decisions which suggests that context is important to how decisions are made as well as the knowledge and expertise used to make them. Thus, an expert professional is not a commodity which can be transferred between areas or specialities without thought. An expert nurse is an expert in their field, and their greatest value lies therein. This may be problematic where it is expected that following protocols will mean that an individual can follow these equally well in a variety of settings. It is possible that the protocol itself can be followed across settings. However, the ability to make judgements about a patient's multifaceted needs, which should accompany protocol use to ensure appropriate application, will not necessarily be transferable.

QUANTIFICATION AND EXPERTISE

This book has consistently identified that financial considerations are a reality of healthcare. Expert practitioners are often a costly commodity, and the need to account for cost applies equally to the value attributed to expert practice as to other areas of healthcare. Smith (2003) suggests that unless the value of something can be measured it is likely to be unattractive to managers, who must account for their spending. Although the introduction of national clinical guidelines and care protocols has the intention of promoting high-quality care, they equally have cost-containment agendas. While expertise in healthcare practice is said to be valued, and indeed one of the aims of government policy is said to be to reward expertise (DoH, 2000), how the unquantifiable nature of expert judgement fits the drive towards standardisation, measurable achievement and quantifiable efficiency is problematic. For expertise to be valued, and for the cost of expert staff, rather than competent staff who can follow clinical guidelines or care protocols, to be accepted as necessary, healthcare staff must be able to articulate the value of their expertise. This may be problematic, as the nature of expertise, particularly in nursing, means that the decisions made are often unquantifiable.

Johnson and Hauser (2001) describe how expert nurses in psychiatric settings 'deescalate violence in patients'. The narratives from their accounts identify the aspects of their thinking which achieve this and explain how experts act to prevent violent episodes from occurring. However, although how decisions are made and adverse incidents avoided can be described, it may not be possible to measure how effective this was, for example how many violent incidents such experts avert compared to less expert practitioners. The fact that these incidents are avoided makes them difficult to quantify. In addition, expert staff are likely to care for the less well or less stable patients, which may in fact skew results to suggest that experts have poorer outcomes.

Despite the difficulty of quantifying expertise, it seems expedient for health-care staff to consider how they can articulate and justify the cost of expert staff. This will include considering how they will be able to justify qualitative aspects of care in a world where quantification may be the priority, and how they can explain the value of expertise. It may be possible to quantify the effect of expertise, for example by recording the estimated level of risk of violence for each patient cared for, whether 'expert' or 'non-expert' nurses cared for each and how each group scored in relation to risk of violence and actual violence. However, this may be problematic to actually record, and in many cases the nature of the outcomes of expert care will not be so obvious. The nature of expertise means that narrative accounts and a naturalistic, not positivist, approach will usually be needed to explain and justify expert decision-making. This may be achieved by using case studies which illustrate the concept of expert decision-making and show how this is distinct from experience or following protocols. Comparisons with concepts such as fuzzy logic which are based in the 'scientific' world and therefore suggest that even those whose focus is usually quantification accept that this is inadequate to explain expertise may also be useful. Nevertheless, the likely conflict between the way in which expert decision-making can best be explained and the predominantly positivist world of clinical guidelines and care protocols, in which generalisability is the intention, is one which healthcare professionals should be aware of so as to be prepared for this type of debate.

DEVELOPING EXPERTISE AND CLINICAL GUIDELINES AND CARE PROTOCOLS

There has been some concern expressed that, as well as reducing the value of expert judgement, the use of clinical guidelines and care protocols will stifle the development of expertise as staff will learn to follow these, rather than to develop clinical decision-making skills. The DoH (2002) claim that using care protocols will increase the autonomy of certain professional groups by enabling them to expand their role remit and thus provide holistic care. Nevertheless, if the provision of care using prespecified care protocols or clinical guidelines, rather than the provision of holistic care, becomes the focus, there may be a return to a situation akin to the task-allocation approach which nursing at least has moved away from. A range of staff may be seen as able to follow given protocols to carry out individual aspects of care for each patient, but this may not mean that one individual provides holistic and expert care that meets the whole needs of the person. How clinical guidelines and care protocols are used will therefore, to a great extent, determine whether they result in expert holistic or task-orientated, fragmented care. They have the potential to do either.

Whether staff learn to regard clinical guidelines and care protocols as tools to be used to aid decision-making and the provision of holistic care or as rigid rules to be followed across the board is in part determined by how these tools are used in preparation for practice and in continuing professional development. Care protocols and clinical guidelines may be useful tools for education, to structure and facilitate learning about given conditions or approaches to treatment and care. The steps outlined may be discussed in relation to why this is recommended, how recommended steps link to pathophysiology, psychology and pharmacology, and thus they may be used to provide case-related, clinically relevant teaching and to show how theory links to practice. It is also possible to structure teaching around guidelines or protocols to facilitate discussion of why certain recommendations are made and what the alternatives are, so as to foster familiarity with identifying and using evidence to inform practice and a questioning approach in which guidelines and protocols are not blindly accepted.

However, in order to avoid the development of a generation of healthcare staff who are simply protocol- or guideline-driven caregivers, staff also need to develop expert decision-making skills. This means students being exposed to the skills and knowledge involved in expert decision-making in practice and discussing and observing how clinical guidelines and care protocols can be a part, but not the entirety of, professional decision-making. Developing expertise involves learning theory, but must also embrace practice-based education. There is general agreement that expert decision-making draws on a vast range of knowledge, experience and skills (Radwin, 1995; Rolfe, 1996; King and Clark, 2002; Martin, 2000). Understanding this type of decision-making is important, but such analysis is generally carried out subconsciously, almost instantaneously, continuously and often in a busy environment. It can therefore be difficult for novice staff to learn from their expert colleagues, as the time needed to explain and explore expert decision-making is not often available. Practice-based education staff may be able to facilitate the development of such discussions, with students or trained staff, so that how experts make decisions can be understood and developed (Maiden and Hewitt-Taylor, 2005). This includes illustrating situations where protocols or guidelines were followed and where it was decided that this was not in the patient's best interests.

SUMMARY

Clinical guidelines and care protocols should repesent a summary of recommendations based on the current best evidence. However, this does not obviate a practitioner's legal and professional responsibility to use their clinical judgement to determine the best course of action in each individual situation.

Clinical guidelines and care protocols are intended to guide and facilitate, but not replace, clinical decision-making (Considine and Hood, 2000). Expert practice may include the use of care protocols or clinical guidelines, but experts will decide, in each situation, whether a guideline or protocol is appropriate for use. They will assimilate the information included in guidelines or protocols along with their previous experience, knowledge, skills and intuitive judgement to make and effect appropriate, rapid decisions.

One risk in a healthcare system in which cost is a very real consideration and finite resources must be used for the good of all is that acceptable but fragmented and protocol-driven care may be seen as more cost-effective than expert, holistic care. Healthcare professionals may therefore need to not only develop clinical expertise but to be able to articulate clearly how expert practice enhances care.

There is a potential problem that, if care protocols or clinical guidelines become the normal approach to care provision, care will become stagnant. NICE state that their guideline development programme is intended to facilitate innovation as well as other factors (NICE, 2005b). However, an overdependence on existing guidelines and protocols may mean that patients who could benefit from unusual treatment will not be offered it, or new approaches cannot be developed because it is perceived that guidelines or protocols must be followed. There is thus a risk that, far from reducing care based on tradition and habit, clinical guidelines and care protocols may themselves become a form of ritual or tradition-based practice.

One intention of guidelines and protocols is to protect the public from cavalier approaches to experimental treatment (Kennedy, 2001). There is, nonetheless, a place for debating when the opportunity for individuals to receive care or treatment options which are outside the scope of guidelines or protocols is advantageous to them and potentially to future patients, provided they are adequately informed about this and the risks involved (Wolfson *et al.*, 2005).

9
Patient Choice

National clinical guidelines and care protocols aim to make recommendations based on the current best evidence of the clinical efficacy and cost-effectiveness of treatment, interventions or care processes. Their intention is also to increase the equality of standards of healthcare which individuals receive, regardless of their geographical location (DoH, 2002). The DoH, nonetheless, state that clinical guidelines and care protocols should be used in a way that is sensitive to individual need and that patients should have more choice over their treatment and care than has traditionally been the case (DoH, 1998). Likewise, the Bristol Inquiry (Kennedy, 2001) encouraged healthcare staff to pay increased attention to patients' views and to improve their involvement in decision-making. It also recommended the production of clear national guidance on what treatment or care patients can expect to receive from the NHS. Thus, at a national level, there is a requirement to increase patients' involvement in healthcare and enhance their choice and a recommendation that individuals and organisations should concurrently adhere to certain national standards of practice.

Although this may mean that patients receive equal standards of specific elements of care covered by clinical guidelines or care protocols, it may be difficult to jointly achieve the use of pre-specified guidelines or protocols and patient choice. This chapter therefore discusses the congruence or other-wise of clinical guidelines and care protocols with patients having improved choices about their healthcare and being more involved in health-related decision-making.

THE IDEAL OF PATIENT INVOLVEMENT AND CHOICE

Respecting patients' rights to make decisions about their health and seeing them as partners in decision-making are high on the current professional and political agendas (Joffe *et al.*, 2003; Sullivan, 2003). The RCN's (2003) definition of nursing places partnership between nurse and patient, charac-

terised by negotiation and patient empowerment, centrally. The GMC also
state that one of the three main responsibilities of doctors is to respect patient
autonomy (GMC, 2005).

The recognition of patients' understanding of, and contribution to, the management of their own health and an increased regard for patient autonomy is
a significant change from the stance which historically permeated healthcare.
Traditionally, medical staff were seen as knowing what was in a patient's best
interests and making decisions accordingly (Kennedy, 2003). This paternalistic stance included acceptance that medical staff would make decisions about
treatment and care on behalf of patients, without necessarily ascertaining their
views or preferences. It also meant medical staff having the therapeutic priv-
ilege to withhold information if they felt that this would be in a patient's best
interests. This was seen at the time as being appropriate and not detrimental
to a patient's well-being. Kennedy (2003) identifies that, on the contrary, it was
considered unreasonable and even harmful to impose the burden of decision-
making on patients. The expectation of individuals and society was that
patients would be told by healthcare staff what their needs were and how these
would be met. Hewitt (2002) suggests that this traditional medical paternalism resulted in patients being in a position in which they felt unequal and disinclined to question medical decision-making. This in turn perpetrated the
view that patients were unable to make decisions regarding their healthcare
and should rely on professionals for this and the expectation by patients that
this would happen. An absence of need or opportunity to make decisions not
only means you do not make decisions but also means you lose your tendency
and inclination to do so, and your confidence that you can.

When my partner and I went trekking in the Sahara, we needed guides,
because wandering about the desert in the same vacant way as I wander about
a Greyhound bus station is not such a good idea – and Ordnance Survey maps
of the Sahara are hard to come by. For seven days, we were completely at their
mercy. They told us when to get up, presented us with our food and drinks,
told us when to set off, whether we should ride or walk and accompanied us
every step of the way. Because we were on unfamiliar territory, and communication was a little stilted and mostly in French, we did as we were told. We
drank hideous green tea without argument and ate petrol-flavoured biscuits
because that is what, amongst other tastier things, we were given. On the first
day, it was strange to be so dependent, but by the fourth day it no longer
occurred to us that we might make a decision, because that was not what we
did. We couldn't decide the route because we had no idea of the directions.
However, we could have declined the petrol-flavoured biscuits. There was
enough other food available, but, at the end of the day's hike, to sustain me
until we ate tagine, I would be presented with and indulge in a couple of petrol
delicacies. It may be the same with healthcare. Even individuals who are able
to make decisions without any difficulty in other walks of life may find this

hard if they are unused to healthcare situations and if the expectation is that they will comply with what healthcare staff say.

Although the paternalistic model of healthcare persisted for many years, it is now generally seen as an unhelpful approach to health-related decision-making (Kennedy, 2003). It is also viewed as unethical and potentially damaging to a patient's well-being to fail to provide them with full information about their health, treatment and care and involve them in decision-making, as this impairs their autonomy.

Respect for autonomy is arguably the most fundamental of moral principles (Fletcher and Buka, 1999), and respect for patient autonomy could therefore be described as one of the most fundamental moral requirements of healthcare professionals. Ethics and morals are intrinsically linked, an ethic being defined as 'a set of moral principles' (Oxford English Dictionary, 2001) and ethics as 'the moral principles governing or influencing conduct' (Oxford English Dictionary, 2001). Respecting autonomy is one of the four main aspects of medical ethics, but also links with the other ethical principles of healthcare. Healthcare professionals are required to fulfil the ethical obligations to do good (beneficence) and to do no harm (non-maleficence), and how the promotion of patient autonomy links with the requirement to do good and avoid harm is therefore also a consideration in healthcare ethics. It has been suggested that reducing a person's autonomy reduces their well-being and that a failure to respect autonomy thus not only means that the ethical requirement to respect autonomy is breached but also means that the principles of beneficence and non-maleficence are not met (Wilmot, 2003). From this perspective, it seems that promoting autonomy is an indisputable part of healthcare and that any other stance is morally and ethically reprehensible. This brings into question why, for such a long period of time, healthcare professionals saw acting in a paternalistic manner as acceptable.

It has been suggested that this was seen as acceptable because of an argument that as an individual's level of autonomy is improved by having good physical health, and thus that a temporary infringement of their autonomy in relation to healthcare decision-making was morally permissible if this had the aim of improving their physical health and therefore, by implication, ultimately their autonomy (Wilmot, 2003). However, Wilmot suggests that, although this argument has been used, it is not generally a justifiable approach and that other issues are involved when healthcare staff choose to make decisions on behalf of adults who have not been deemed incapable of exercising their autonomy. This is no longer an argument which is generally accepted in healthcare as a justification for excluding patients from decision-making.

The principle of justice is the fourth major principle of medical ethics, and how this interfaces with autonomy will be discussed later in this chapter, and in Chapter 10. However, in some respects these two principles may be hard to reconcile in a healthcare system where funding is finite and resources must be used justly, for the good of all. The principle of justice has the intention of ensuring that all individuals have equal access to what might be considered a basic commodity, such as healthcare (Wilmot, 2003). However, this is not as easy to achieve as it might seem as it includes taking into account the availability of local and national resources and the vast range of health-related needs for which finite funding must be used (Fletcher and Buka, 1999; Bridges *et al.*, 2001). As the medical and technological capacity to manage increasingly complex health needs has expanded, so too have dilemmas over resource allocation. The funds and other resources which are available to meet the ever-increasing need or potential to provide care are finite and often inadequate to meet all the demands placed upon them (Boosfeld and O'Toole, 2000; Poses, 2003). Patient choice cannot, therefore, be absolute, and autonomy in this situation cannot include having absolute choice. It means choice within real-world limits.

WHY PATIENT CHOICE AND AUTONOMY IS PROMOTED

Despite the ethical imperative to promote autonomy, there may be reasons other than healthcare staff recognising the importance of promoting patient autonomy in the current move towards patient involvement in decision-making. Gallant *et al.* (2002) suggest that the development of a recognition of the need for an equal relationship between patients and healthcare staff has occurred because of an increase in democratic thinking in society as a whole, not just in healthcare. In British culture individuals are now generally more aware of their rights, and expect to have choices. This applies equally to their health as to other aspects of their lives (Kennedy, 2003). It is therefore not just, and in some cases not principally, the result of changes in attitudes in healthcare or a desire on the part of healthcare staff to honour patient autonomy which has led to the recognition of a need for greater involvement of patients in decision-making. Rather, it is a reflection of changes in society as a whole.

The need for healthcare professionals to discuss, not dictate, care options has also become a necessity in a society in which deference is no longer unquestioningly given to professionals, including healthcare staff (Wilmot, 2003). British society is no longer one in which a physician's view will necessarily be accepted simply because they are a physician.

A contributory factor to the change in perceptions of healthcare providers may have been well-publicised cases of misconduct, and instances where healthcare professionals and organisations have fallen short of the standards which the public might expect of them (Canter, 2001). Cases such as Beverly Allitt (Clothier, 1994), Harold Shipman (Smith, 2005) and the Bristol Inquiry (Kennedy, 2001) have indicated that it cannot always be assumed that healthcare staff have their patients' best interests at heart and that, even when they have, this will not always mean that what they do is in fact the best thing for their patients. There have also been more general concerns over standards of healthcare, for example rates of hospital-acquired infection. In addition, the legal right of healthcare professionals to decide about the care of individual patients has been publicly challenged (Dyer, 2004), and the legal evidence given by Roy Meadow (Dyer, 2005) found to be inaccurate to a vastly damaging degree. This combination of events, it is argued, have resulted in patients no longer feeling able to unquestioningly accept the views of healthcare professionals.

There are also potential benefits for organisations if they apparently increase patient involvement in care decisions. The government now include patient feedback in star ratings (Coulter, 2002), and patient satisfaction as well as the medical outcomes of treatment and the meeting of targets are therefore likely to be important in how NHS Trusts are rated, which has organisational and financial implications. As well as seeking to develop respectful relationships with patients because this is ethically and morally 'right', NHS Trusts may need to be seen to treat patients with respect in order to gain good feedback and retain financial and managerial independence.

Although there is sometimes a fear that patient choice will be costly, paternalistic approaches to treatment may be more costly. Coulter (2002) suggests that paternalism does little to foster self-reliance. As self-reliance in relation to health is likely to decrease dependence on healthcare staff, and thus reduce service use, it may be more cost-effective to promote patient self-management than to encourage reliance on healthcare staff.

Thus, although there may be a genuine desire to promote patient autonomy amongst healthcare staff, it would be simplistic to think that this change from the approach which has historically permeated healthcare has occurred simply because of professionals deciding that patient autonomy is intrinsically good and should be respected.

In addition, although this is the current trend in healthcare, achieving a true shift in power, and a change in the beliefs and values of individual professionals and professions as a whole, is not easy to achieve (Canter, 2001). An entire profession or professions are unlikely, overnight, to achieve an about-turn in how they view patient involvement in decision-making. If they appear to do so, or are required to do so, there is a risk that this will not be a true change but rather a superficial acceptance of the party line, with individuals' actual beliefs and values unchanged. Paternalism is a culture in which medicine, and to some degree healthcare in general, has spent many years. Tweedale (2002) argues that, despite apparent changes in ethos, latent paternalism is likely to surface when staff are asked by patients to follow a course of action which is in conflict with their own perspective. It is fairly easy to allow patients choice and involvment, and to respect patients' views when these coincide with the ideas of healthcare professionals, but the true test of whether autonomy is respected is how professionals respond when patients choose a path which does not coincide with their views.

In addition, the complexity of promoting true patient autonomy is not something that should be underestimated, and understanding this is necessary if it is to be achieved.

AUTONOMY

Promoting and sustaining patient autonomy may be more difficult to enact than is often suggested. It requires considerable effort by healthcare staff, including time, motivation and insight into one's own atttitudes and values and how these affect interactions with patients.

Autonomy is defined as an individual's ability to make self-determining choices and involves the individual having independence, the capacity to reason and the ability to make decisions (Lowden, 2002). To be autonomous, individuals must therefore be independent, be able to take in and consider the various available alternatives and be able to make a decision. To make an autonomous decision about healthcare, patients will therefore need adequate information. An individual may be independent, able to reason and to make decisions, but, in order to make autonomous decisions regarding their health, they need sufficient information.

The distinction should be made between an individual's ability to function autonomously, and healthcare professionals' skills in conveying information in an appropriate manner and their ability and willingness to listen to patients' views and questions (Lowden, 2002). For example, a surgeon being unable to explain in terms which a family can understand the implications of their child having a certain type of cardiac surgery does not necessarily mean that the family lack the intrinsic ability to be autonomous. It may rather mean that the surgeon lacks communication skills. A person with special communication needs may require explanations to be made using communication devices or systems which healthcare staff are unfamiliar with. However, this again does not mean they are not, of themselves, capable of functioning autonomously. It means that healthcare staff need to increase their range of communication skills, and to plan their interactions so that someone who can act as 'interpreter' and use the appropriate communication devices can be present to facilitate information-giving.

In our Saharan sojourn, we could, technically, have made choices, but we had not much information and were on seriously unfamiliar territory. This situation was augmented by the language deficit. I speak no Arabic at all; so we communicated mostly in French, Morocco's second language, with occasional bits of English and Spanish, and sometimes a mixture of all three in one sentence. My French is good enough for pleasant conversation about everyday life but doesn't really run to the finer points of navigation in the Sahara and camels. Although I could remember what biscuits were called in French, I unaccountably couldn't think of the term 'petrol-flavoured'; so information exchange was not easy and requesting that the biscuits cease to appear on account of their flavour problematic. This was entirely our fault, because we had made no effort to learn Arabic, but it illustrates the point that, if you are in an unfamiliar situation, lacking information, lacking confidence in the language used and in a culture where you are not expected to question the decisions made on your behalf, being autonomous is not easy.

Even where the intention is to promote autonomy and involve patients, and where staff take considerable trouble to provide substantial information in an appropriate format, Canter (2001) suggests that decision-making in healthcare generally occurs in an environment in which patients are on unfamiliar territory, receiving information from a traditional biomedical perspective and where this perspective remains unquestioned. Thus, it is unlikely, however well-intentioned healthcare staff are, that patients will easily receive value-free information, even when they receive extensive and comprehensible information. The challenge inherent in giving unbiased information is often described as being problematic because of a biomedical bias. However, it may equally be the case that healthcare staff attempt, albeit with good intentions, to influence patients to follow a non-medical model of care. For example, midwives may promote what is described as 'natural' childbirth with good intentions, but nonetheless present information that is biased by their own and their profession's beliefs and values. This may be in conflict with the preferences of some women and may become problematic where assisted delivery or Caesarean section is in fact necessary and in the infant and woman's best interests. It may result in the woman either delaying consent to Caesarean section or, post delivery, feeling that she did not achieve what was best for her child and thus adversely affect both of their well-beings.

Giving information in a way which facilitates patient autonomy means giving unbiased information. It is difficult to give information without any influence from one's own interpretation of the facts, priorities and beliefs. Canter (2001) identifies that information will almost inevitably be influenced to some degree by the individual practitioner's views of health and their interpretation of the evidence which is available. It is also necessary to consider that what is deemed to be best practice at any point in time may change as new evidence comes to light or as sociey's values and norms change. Healthcare professionals should therefore acknowledge that they do not possess complete and irrefutable knowledge and should adopt a stance from which they and their patients can enter into discussions in which uncertainties and conflicting views can be explored openly (Canter, 2001).

Although autonomy is concerned with self-determination, it does not mean that healthcare staff should leave patients to make decisions in unsupported isolation. An autonomous person can accept support and assistance from others, and can also choose to defer to others. Indeed, a part of healthcare staff's responsibility is to support patients in their decision-making. In addition, Dunn (2002) suggests that although promoting patient involvement in decision-making is curently high on healthcare agendas, not all patients will want to make the final decisions about their care, or, in some cases, be involved in decision-making. Brinchmann *et al.* (2002) found that the parents of premature infants did not generally want to have the final say in decisions regarding continuation or otherwise of their babies' treatment, but that they valued being well informed and listened to during the decision-making process. De Haes and Koedoot (2003) also identify that in palliative care many patients appear to prefer to leave their doctors to make difficult decisions about their treatment. Individuals who have been used to medical staff making decisions on their behalf for many years, for example the elderly, may not in fact wish to change this, however much society as a whole may see this as the best course of action. Autonomous decision-making includes individuals being self-determining in deciding how far they wish to be involved in decisions (Kaplan, 2002). However, where a patient allows healthcare staff to make decisions on their behalf, staff should be clear that this is a choice by the patient, not a fait accompli by healthcare professionals or a situation in which the patient feels unable to question the decisions of healthcare staff or enter into discussion with them (Lowden, 2002).

DECISION-MAKING IN AN UNCERTAIN WORLD

Many decisions in healthcare do not have clear 'right' or 'wrong' answers. Thus, no one but the individual who is affected by it can determine what is a good or bad outcome. The extent to which an intervention, treatment, aspect of care provision or outcome of care is beneficial or harmful is affected by the values which individual patients hold (Protheroe *et al.*, 2000; O'Connor *et al.*, 2004). Thus, patient involvement in decision-making is necessary because healthcare staff, despite possibly knowing scientific variables and how patients in a broadly similar situation have responded do not know each individual's circumstances, values and priorities. Protheroe *et al.* (2000) found that medical staff tend to view an intervention's success in relation to the extent of symptom control, technical success or physiological parameters, while patients measure the success of an intervention in terms of its effect on their general health and life quality. Therefore, to achieve good decisions for individuals the perspectives of those individuals must be included. For example, a patient who has a life-threatening illness may have a specific goal – to see their grandchild born, to attend their son's wedding – or to achieve a lifetime desire, for example to see the Grand Canyon. Such goals may supersede any desire for longevity and may influence their decisions about the relative risks and benefits of treatment options.

Coulter (2002) suggests that medical staff should be well informed and able to give advice on diagnostics, disease processes, prognosis and treatment but that only the patient knows their experience of illness, their social circumstances, habits, behaviours, attitudes to risk, values and preferences. Both types of knowledge are needed in healthcare decision-making as all these factors will affect whether an outcome is good for an individual. However, despite Coulter (2002) suggesting that medical staff should be in possession of knowledge about diseases, treatments and interventions, the division of knowledge between healthcare pofessionals and patients may not be so clearcut as this suggests. There are many situations in which there is scientific uncertainty over the effectiveness of treatment (O'Connor *et al.*, 2004). Thus, healthcare staff may not be able to state with absolute certainty the medical or physical outcomes even though they may be able to state their knowledge of the current best evidence. In addition, in some situations patients may have more medical or technical information than healthcare staff. Chapters 1 and 3 identified the changes in the volume and quality of health-related information available to the public, the pros and cons of this and how it affects the drive towards evidence-based practice. However, the vast range of information which is available, and the ever-increasing spectrum of disease and treatment options means that healthcare professionals often face an almost impossible task to be aware of all the information in all areas of their field of practice. In addition, the speed with which knowledge develops and is presented, for example electronic dissemination, means that patients who have a given condition may access a greater volume of more current information than healthcare professionals. Thus, although the usual assumption is that healthcare staff know more about the medical and technical aspects of health and illness than patients, this may not always be the case.

Thus, the knowledge, experience, values and beliefs of healthcare staff and patients all need to be included in effective, shared decision-making about what will be best in individual cases (O'Connor *et al.*, 2004; Hu *et al.*, 2004). Although this is the ideal, it requires healthcare staff to be prepared to engage in such debates, to feel confident in facilitating this type of discussion and to be able to assist patients to use the information which has been discussed to weigh up the pros and cons of any given care option. This may be daunting for many staff and may contribute to a reluctance to enter into such debates.

DECISION-MAKING TOOLS

To facilitate patient involvement in decision-making there needs to be good communication between health professionals and patients. However, given the complexities involved in decision-making, there is a need for staff to have more than a desire to involve patients and good general communication skills. They need strategies for explaining the existing evidence and guidance, its stengths and limitations, and the boundaries of choice. They also need the ability to facilitate discussion of how these points fit with the individual's priorities, beliefs and values and how any divergence can be best managed. This type of discussion will also include acknowledging the inherent uncertainty of many healthcare situations (Griffiths *et al.*, 2005). This can make assisting patients to achieve autonomous choices a daunting prospect.

There are tools in existence whose aim is to assist practitioners to structure and conduct such discussions and to assist patients to be clear about what their preferences are. O'Connor *et al.* (2004) describe the use of evidence-based 'patient decision' aids as an adjunct to practitioners communicating with patients. These tools include information on the available options, the relative risks of interventions or treatment, the likely outcomes, probabilities and scientific uncertainties. They also include various tools to assist patients to clarify and communicate the personal value which they place on the various risks or benefit-versus-harm aspects of the interventions in question. The intention is therefore that the clinical and personal aspects of decision-making are covered so that the best decision for individuals can be reached and so that patients and healthcare staff have a clear understanding of why the decision in question was reached. These tools are not intended to replace staff–patient interaction but rather to facilitate the process and to give both parties tools to guide what can be complex and difficult discussions. They may be self-administered to prepare patients for discussions, or practitioner-administered at the time of consultation. Protheroe (2000) also describes a form of computerised decision analysis tool that compares the probability of outcomes of treatment and incorporates estimates of patients' perceptions of the consequences of treatment and the values and priorities which they place on the various potential outcomes. In both cases, as is important in healthcare decision-making, patients' values and priorities are included rather than simply the likelihood or otherwise of medical or technical success determined by physiological outcomes.

THE LIMITS OF CHOICE WITHIN FINITE RESOURCES

Although the aim of current government policy is to increase patient choice, this is not necessarily easy to achieve alongside other considerations in a nationally resourced health service. The GMC (2000) and NMC (2002) acknowledge that while medical and nursing staff should provide care which takes account of patients' preferences this must be within the limits of finite resources. Although the focus is often on assisting patients to achieve a decision about what is best for them, this belies the broader context of patient choice. For individual patients the right decision is the one which maximises their well-being, but in a resource-constrained healthcare system this will not always coincide with the right decision for patients in general and society as a whole (Wailoo *et al.*, 2004).

The ethical principle of justice may be difficult to reconcile with the principle of individual autonomy as choice cannot be absolute in a healthcare system where central resources, funded by public money, must be used for the good of all. Grace (2001) identifies that actions taken in relation to the care of one patient necessarily have implications beyond that patient. Choices made by one patient will also affect other patients. Although justice is sometimes seen as meaning that all patients will have their needs equally met, this may be unrealistic where the resources available are outstripped by the demand for healthcare. The aim of government policy is necessarily likely to be to achieve good health for all population groups and the best care for the greatest number of people, not equal healthcare provision for all individuals (Kazanjian, 2001). Utilitarian principles are often used to justify decisions about how best to use limited public funds, that is what will be the most productive use of resources and the greatest good for the greatest number of individuals (Draper and Sorell, 2002). This may be a useful premise, but given the differing views on what constitutes health and the priorities which individuals have within this, what is considered beneficial or harmful is difficult to determine for entire populations. Deciding what is the 'greatest good' for the greatest number may therefore be problematic. Nevertheless, judging an action solely on the benefit of its own outcome, isolated from broader consequences, is often considered incompatible with the complexities of modern healthcare in which decisions made in relation to one patient will inevitably impact on the resources available for others.

This need to consider the entire picture of healthcare as well as individual need includes taking into account the time needed to fully involve patients in decision-making and how this impacts upon the time available for other aspects of care and the care of other patients (Dunn, 2002). Involving patients in decision-making is now usually seen as an essential part of care, but the facilitation of decision-making for one patient impacts on the time which staff have to enable other patients to make high-quality decisions. The resources available to facilitate informed decision-making are therefore also finite. There are no easy answers to how these points should be balanced, but they are factors which healthcare staff and patients should be aware of. Autonomy does not equal unlimited choice. Rather, it means decision-making within real-world limitations.

PATIENT AUTONOMY AND RESPONSIBILITY

The reality of the resources available for healthcare provision being finite and choices therefore being limited is a part of the information which should be available to patients if they are to make truly informed decisions (GMC, 2000). If patients are autonomous, and not vulnerable individuals who must be protected from the onus of decision-making by medical paternalism, they must also be seen as able to function in the real world, in which the finite nature of healthcare resources is a part of reality. They must also be seen as responsible as autonomy comes hand in hand with responsibility (Draper and Sorell, 2002). A part of autonomy is therefore being aware that, within a healthcare system which is publicly funded and free at the point of delivery there are limits on choice, that they are responsible for the choices which they make and that the choices which they make affect others.

There has therefore been a suggestion that individuals who knowingly engage in lifestyles or activities which may damage their health should not have the same access to free care to resolve such damage as those who have not knowingly engaged in such activities (Draper and Sorell, 2002). One problem in this argument is deciding what would be seen as acceptable or unacceptable risk-taking by patients. Risk factors in healthcare can be defined as behaviours, conditions, inherited traits or lifestyle choices that increase a person's chances of developing a disease, or of that disease deteriorating. Some of these factors can be modified, treated or controlled but some cannot (Muminovic, 2002; Edwards et al., 2002). However, there are a vast range of risk factors which exist and the complexity of interactions between aspects of an individual's biological makeup and lifestyle mean that it is problematic to determine how decisions regarding what risk was seen as acceptable or otherwise would be reached. One of the focuses in the proposed limitations on healthcare was obesity, with the suggestion that individuals who were obese and failed to reduce their body weight should have limitations on healthcare provision for illnesses related to obesity. However, this has the potential to become a judgement based on society's values and prejudices, not responsibility. There was, for example, no suggestion that individuals who were injured in high-impact or dangerous sports should be excluded. If I were injured climbing in the Andes, provided my insurers would repatriate me, there was no suggestion that my irresponsible chosen leisure activity, which is entirely within my control to participate in or not, would be deemed unworthy of treatment. Given the multifaceted nature of health, and the need to consider social, emotional, psychological, spiritual and physical well-being, decisions about risk and adverse effects on health are problematic and open to value judgements which would be hard to justify. Draper and Sorell (2002) acknowledge that this is problematic and that behaviour alone is also a crude measure of risk, with genetic and environmental factors also contributing to health outcomes. However, what is clear is that autonomy is not without responsibility and that, for healthcare staff to meaningfully engage in promoting patient autonomy and partnership in decision-making, discussions may need to include the more problematic aspects of autonomy such as limits on resources and one individual's responsibility to others.

GUIDELINES, PROTOCOLS AND PATIENT CHOICES

The place which clinical guidelines and care protocols occupy in the debate on patient choice relates largely to the fact that patients should know what is available to them, what is recommended and why, and that choice in a publicly funded healthcare system is not absolute. Clinical guidelines and care protocols may be a double-edged sword. They may make explicit to patients what is available, what they can expect and why. This may be helpful for patients as they will know the menu of options from which they can choose and may be helpful for practitioners as a tool to frame debates over the available choices. It may also make clear that where there are limitations on choice this is not the random decision of individual practitioners but central decision-making over the use of resources. However, the downside of clinical guidelines and care protocols in relation to patient choice is that they make explicit recommendations, which practitioners may be reluctant or unable to deviate from, thus reducing choice. This is likely to be particularly marked where relatively expensive treatments are in question and patients would choose to receive, rather than decline, them.

Smeeth (2000) suggests patient choices for treatment often disagree with consensual guidelines and guidelines based on an assessment of absolute risk. This is often interpreted as meaning that allowing patients choice is a negative financial approach as it will be an expensive option. However, this will not always be the case. Protheroe *et al.* (2002) suggests that in the case of patients who are being treated for atrial fibrillation, taking into account patient preferences would mean that fewer patients were prescribed warfarin than under published guideline recommendations thus reducing the cost of treatment.

The extent to which clinical guidelines or care protocols affect patient choice will be largely dependent upon how much duress is attached to the guideline or protocol being adhered to both nationally and locally. This includes the duress under which organisations are placed to follow clinical guidelines or care protocols and the degree of duress under which individual practitioners perceive themselves to be placed. For example, if an obstetrician feels under duress to avoid performing Caesarean sections, it is likely to adversely affect the extent to which they truly facilitate women making informed choices.

Many of the points which have been made about patient involvement in decision-making hold true regardless of the existence or otherwise of care protocols or clinical guidelines. The difference is that, where specifics are set, debates will emanate from these and not from individual practitioner views.

This may be a positive step, in so far as there is less chance of individual practitioners' personal biases affecting patient choice. However, it means that individuals and organisations may be under, or perceive themselves to be under, duress to follow clinical guidelines and care protocols rather than engaging in the process of shared decision-making.

Clinical guidelines and care protocols may therefore both facilitate and impede elements of patient choice. They are, however, a current reality of healthcare and therefore a part of the real world in which patients must make decisions.

10

Finite Resources, Infinite Demand

Clinical guidelines and care protocols are intended to enhance the quality, but also the cost-effectiveness, of patient care. Cost is therefore something that has to be considered in discussions about developing and using clinical guidelines and care protocols.

Cost is an increasingly important consideration in all aspects of healthcare. In a publicly funded health service, such as the NHS, which is free to users at the point of delivery, the needs of the entire population as well as the needs of individuals must be considered. This can be seen at the level of direct care, where the time taken by a nurse to provide care for one patient affects the time available for them to provide care for others. It also applies at a wider level in relation to what funds are available and how these will be spent. For example, the cost of providing intensive treatment and care to save the life of a premature baby born at 23 weeks' gestation is considerable, and must be taken from a central resource that is intended to provide care for all.

The medical and technological capacity to preserve life and treat ill health has expanded significantly since the inception of the NHS. At the same time, there have been considerable developments in preventative medicine and public health. This means that unless there is a significant rise in taxation decisions must be made as to how finite healthcare resources will be used to meet what is effectively an infinite demand. This inevitably leads to the need for some form of rationing of healthcare for the population as a whole, as the potential to treat outstrips the financial ability to provide immediate intervention for all these options. It also means that healthcare professionals cannot expect to work in ivory towers detached from the reality of the cost of care.

Despite the inevitability of cost affecting healthcare provision, and the fact that cost is a consideration in healthcare, the idea of care being rationed and of cost forming a major consideration in healthcare is often uncomfortable for healthcare professionals and the public. The direct-care relationship between a patient and their healthcare provider has meant that traditionally what is best for that individual has been the professional's prime, if not only, concern. However, the reality of a publicly funded health service is that the cost of one patient's treatment impacts on what is available for others and that this affects every level of decision-making from ward level to government level.

One reason for the development of national clinical guidelines is to address some of the perceived inequality in the provision of healthcare across regions and between healthcare providers (DoH, 2000). The intention is that all individuals in the population should have access to the same range of care options and that there will be clarity over what is available and what it is reasonable for individuals to expect to receive from state healthcare. They are not, therefore, intended to give everything to everyone, but to recommend what should and should not be universally available.

National clinical guidelines must therefore take cost into account. NICE's remit includes considering whether various health-related interventions can be recommended as a use of NHS resources (Rawlins *et al.*, 2001). SIGN also include commentary on the resource implications of their recommendations if these are significant (SIGN, 2004a). Cost is not the only factor that NICE or SIGN consider, neither should it be the overriding one, but resources are an issue which they do not attempt to avoid. One of the major remits of NICE is to provide information and advice on the quality of care that an individual can expect, and this includes providing information on what options for healthcare an individual can expect to be available, and on decisions which have been made in relation to resource allocation (Littlejohns *et al.*, 2004).

THE PRINCIPLES OF HEALTHCARE ECONOMICS

The demand for healthcare is increasing as the understanding of causation of disease and thus methods of early detection and prevention thereof develop. At the same time, the ability to treat life-threatening illness continues to expand. These developments in the ability to prevent ill health and to manage increasingly complex health problems have significant resource implications. Life expectancy is also rising at both ends of the age spectrum. Premature babies can now be treated and sustained at a gestational age which has previously been considered non-viable and life expectancy for the healthy population has increased. Thus, as well as both ends of the population's age spectrum expanding, both ends of the health spectrum – the prevention of ill health and the management of increasingly complex health problems – have developed. With the development of every area of healthcare, dilemmas over resource allocation have inevitably increased (Boosfeld and O'Toole, 2000; Poses, 2003).

Healthcare in the United Kingdom is free at the point of delivery, but publicly funded through taxation and national insurance contributions. Thus, although any treatment and care provided is free to the individual when it is given, it has a cost, which is met by citizens. Although there is no charge levied for each individual healthcare encounter, the cost of meeting the health needs or demands of each individual are taken from a central resource which must be used for all. This means that improvements in one area of healthcare provision are likely to impact on other areas, unless there is no cost involved in the improvement in service. For example, reducing waiting times for some interventions or in some specialities is likely to mean that other areas have a compensatory fall in service unless additional funding is provided. If additional funding is provided, this must either be levied from taxation or taken from another area of public money. Improvements in service may, of course, be achieved without cost, for example if a less expensive drug is found to be more effective than a more costly one, or where advances in surgical techniques mean that patients have reduced duration of pre- and postoperative hospitalisation. However, where additional funding is needed to improve a service, the resources must be taken from somewhere.

As well as the impact of the cost of individual on corporate healthcare, the money used for healthcare also affects the funds available for other areas of public expenditure, such as education and housing. The decisions reached regarding healthcare provision, and what will or will not be provided, therefore have an impact beyond healthcare, to other aspects of public service. In some cases, the impact of health interventions will have a direct impact on other services. For example, advances in medicine and technology mean that there is an increasing population of children with complex and continuing health needs. The cost of their care will include the cost of initial life-saving treatment, ongoing medical and technical interventions, care staff and staff education. It may also include the provision of special housing and special education. While these are all necessary expenses to maximise quality of life for the child and family, this type of provision is costly and spans healthcare funding, education funding and housing funding. Caring for children with complex and continuing needs in the community setting is relatively less costly than providing care in hospital, as well as being in the child's best interests. However, the cost is still significant and affects a wide range of public-funding streams.

Healthcare professionals have traditionally been distanced from considering the financial cost of their decisions, and have often appeared to see such considerations as unethical. However, as decisions made about individual patients have an impact on other patients and society in general, to see patients in isolation is an unrealistic stance. It might also be seen that the failure to consider the resource implications of actions taken in relation to one patient fails to fulfil the duty to act in the best interests of other patients. In addition, given that one of the major principles of medical ethics is justice, it could be seen as unethical not to think beyond the individual patient to how one's actions affect other aspects of healthcare provision. The GMC and NMC both identify that while practitioners should consider the best interests of individual patients this must be within the proviso that they must also consider the good of the population as a whole (GMC, 2005; NMC, 2002).

There is general agreement that it is unrealistic to expect that absolute choice for patients or absolute freedom for practitioners to provide whatever treatment they would prefer can exist where publicly funded resources are used (King's Fund, 2002; GMC, 2000; NMC, 2002). This does not preclude individuals choosing to fund their own healthcare to obtain their choice of intervention, but it is not realistic to think that an organisation such as the NHS can fund everyone's first choice of treatment within the timeframe that they would prefer. Given absolute choice, most staff and patients would prefer to have reduced waiting times for elective surgery, but some waiting times are inevitable and decisions therefore have to be reached over what is a reasonable waiting time for a given intervention. Thus, it is necessary to consider the cost of interventions and the effect which providing this rapidly for some patients will have on the care available for other patients. Reducing waiting times for some procedures or specialities is likely to mean that other areas have a compensatory fall in service unless additional funding is provided. It may also mean that patients are seen more quickly, but for less time, which may reduce the quality of their care despite it being provided more promptly. If additional funding is provided, this must either be levied from taxation or taken from another area of public money.

One approach to reaching such decisions in a manner that is equitable across populations is to provide national guidance on what can and cannot be justified as a reasonable use of resources. The intention of the guidelines issued by NICE and SIGN is to develop national recommendations based on the balance of clinical efficacy and cost-effectiveness on what treatment and care options should be provided, when and by whom.

CALCULATING EFFECTIVENESS

Effectiveness in relation to health in economic terms is generally seen as the extent to which an intervention achieves measurable health improvements, for example cases of disease prevented, years of life saved or quality-adjusted life years saved. Thus, for economic effectiveness to be said to exist, measurement or quantification of outcomes and success is usually deemed to be necessary. Showing that a screening programme increased the detection of early stages of cancer and allowed the instigation of treatment following which there was a high five-year survival rate may demonstrate that this intervention is relatively effective. However, it does not necessarily indicate that it is cost-effective in comparison to other approaches. A method is therefore needed which demonstrates whether or not an intervention is effective in cost terms in comparison to other options.

A method of calculating cost-effectiveness which is often used in healthcare is the incremental cost-effectiveness ratio. The incremental cost of an intervention means the difference between the cost of an intervention and the cost of another intervention, or no intervention, for example the cost of one drug versus the cost of another drug or no drug. The incremental cost-effectiveness ratio is calculated by dividing the incremental cost of an intervention by the incremental effectiveness. Thus, the incremental cost-effectiveness ratio takes into account the overall cost and possible savings of an intervention and therefore produces a calculation on how much of an increase or decrease in overall cost it should produce. Gnafi *et al.* (2004) suggest that this is how NICE calculate the cost-effectiveness of interventions and thus, essentially, this is how NICE make decisions about the financial cost of interventions and whether or not the balance of clinical efficacy and cost-effectiveness makes an intervention worthy of recommendation for use. For example, in their recommendations on the use of bupropion and nicotine replacement therapies, NICE acknowledged that the use of these therapies was initially likely to add some £20–£50 billion to the annual drugs bill in England and Wales. However, they suggested that this would be compensated for by the decrease in spending on smoking-related diseases in the longer term (NICE, 2002f).

An additional challenge in health economics which this raises is the length of time over which savings are calculated. Where short-term budgets are set, and healthcare providers are required to account for spending on an annual or even five-yearly basis, the initial and immediate cost may be all that is seen. The intention to consider long- as well as short-term benefits must be able to be incorporated in budgetary planning as well as the theoretical measuring of health benefits if this model is to be used. For instance, although NICE have calculated that the cost over time of providing smoking-cessation therapies make them cost-effective, if GPs who prescribe this must account for their budgets on a yearly basis, they may have difficulty in justifying this cost regardless of NICE's calculation of the cost-effectiveness ratio.

Although this type of calculation can be used to determine the cost of an intervention, it is also necessary to consider the clinical efficacy of the intervention in order to decide whether the intervention should be used. A drug which can be administered orally may be cheaper than an intravenous drug both in terms of the cost of the drug itself and because it is easily self-administered and reduces those costs associated with hospitalisation or treatment in outpatient departments for intravenous drug administration. However, the savings made by using this approach will be of little actual value if the drug is significantly less effective and results in poor disease control and a greater need for additional treatment and hospitalisation. This still considers cost alone, not quality of life for individual, but the clinical efficacy and cost-effectiveness must both be considered in cost-effectiveness calculations.

Unlike NICE, SIGN do not use this type of formal cost-effectiveness analysis. Their view is that the processes used for economic analysis of healthcare is at a relatively early stage and that although a number of approaches to the incorporation of resource issues into clinical guidelines are under development none is yet considered 'gold standard' (SIGN, 2005). Where there is published economic evidence, this is evaluated and considered alongside other evidence. In cases where there is not published economic evidence on the subject in question, guidelines may include a commentary on the main economic issues that should be considered, for example those found in the SIGN guidelines on hip fracture (SIGN, 2002a) and cardiac rehabilitation (SIGN, 2002b). A final option is for guidelines to include basic information that will allow guideline users to calculate the cost implications for their own service. Examples of this approach can be seen in the SIGN guidelines on osteoporosis (SIGN, 2004b) and epithelial ovarian cancer (SIGN, 2003b).

Any evaluation of the evidence of cost, whichever approach to calculating cost is used, requires consideration of the quality of the data on cost. This includes taking into account the source of information. Miners *et al.* (2005) found that the cost-related information supplied to NICE by manufacturers was significantly more favourable than evaluations produced by academic or research groups, suggesting that bias might exist. The timing of the production of evidence on cost may also be problematic. Stoykova *et al.* (2003) suggest that information on the cost-effectiveness of new treatments may lag behind evidence of their effectiveness. This may mean that a treatment which is not deemed to be cost-effective on published data has in fact become cost-effective or will soon become so. It is also difficult to predict how greater use of a given therapy might increase cost-effectiveness, for example by drug prices being reduced with wider use.

QUALITY

One immediate challenge in estimating the cost versus benefit of an intervention is how to take into account quality of life as well as quantity in determining how effective an intervention is. Economic models are predisposed to quantification, for example increased years of life, reduced episodes of acute exacerbation of disease. However, calculations can also be made that include perceptions of quality of life by developing theoretical trade-offs between quality and quantity of life. For example, time trade-offs may be used whereby it is agreed that a certain number of years without limitations on lifestyle are equal to a greater number of years with severe limitations. For instance, ten years of life with no limitation on mobility might be deemed equal to 25 years of life confined to a wheelchair.

One option which is often used to determine quality of life for populations and to achieve a degree of trade-off between alterations in health state and the cost of interventions is the use of Quality Adjusted Life Years (QALYs). This method assigns a preference weight to each health state and determines the time spent in each state. For instance, ten years with significant limitations may be weighted as being equal to one year with no limitations. To calculate QALYs, the estimate of time spent in each state is used to make a calculation of total quality adjusted life years. This is not total life expectancy but the life years adjusted for what is thought to be quality. For instance, if an individual was expected to live a further 50 years with no limitations or disability, they would have 50 quality adjusted life years. However, if they were expected to live another 50 years with severe limitations which reduced each ten years to only being equivalent to one quality adjusted life year, their QALYs would be five. In weighing up the cost-effectiveness of interventions, QALYs might thus be used to determine effectiveness in quality and quantity terms. If intervention to sustain the life of a critically ill adult would cost £200 000, but was expected to mean that an individual survive 20 additional years, the cost per year would be £10 000. However, if their survival was likely to be with severe limitations, such that their QALYs rather than absolute expected time of survival were only equivalent to four years in good health and without limitation, the cost per QALY would be £50 000. Thus, whereas an estimated annual cost of £10 000 per year might be seen as an acceptable level of cost-effectiveness, a cost of £50 000 might be considered excessive.

Although QALYs are commonly used, they present their own challenges. One problem with the time trade-off method is that unless it is individualised, with discussion of what a limitation on health would mean for an individual, it cannot accurately represent quality issues. For some individuals, life with severely restricted mobility might seem such a burden that they would opt for two years with full mobility rather than 30 years of severely restricted mobility, whereas another individual might not trade any life years overall for it. Thus, making trade-offs in decisions about what will be provided for the population as a whole requires assumptions to be made about what constitutes quality of life, and this differs significantly from person to person. This may be achieved by using consensual views from large population-based studies, so that the perceptions of the majority regarding trade-offs can be made, but it will not mean that the values which are attributed to health states hold true for everyone.

A further problem is that such decisions would usually be taken by individuals before changes in their quality of life occur. The views which people who are in good health have of the theoretical trade-offs which they would make may not be the same as the decisions which they would make were they really required to trade-off life years (Arnsen and Norheim, 2003). Thus, they may not accurately represent how an individual feels about trade-offs when faced with a real situation. For example, a young person who enjoys outdoors adventure activities might feel that five years of being able to continue this lifestyle would be equivalent to 30 with severe limitations of movement. However, if they develop a disease which slowly but progressively affects mobility, their perception of quality of life and the importance which they attach to different aspects of life may alter, and their initial decisions on trade-offs, made when they were well, might not hold.

In addition, as the quality adjustment is overall for populations, and not based on individual perceptions, some groups are likely to be disadvantaged. For example, simply using quality adjusted life years to determine what the spending of the health budget should focus on would potentially mean that treatment for the disabled and elderly would be minimal. A further problem is that QALYs are not considered effective in estimating trade-offs in children as they do not take into account the dynamics of child development and do not include health state classification instruments for use in children younger than five years. A further problem is that QALYs only take into account the health of the child for the child, not the health effects on parents of being parents and of the state of health of their child (Griebsch *et al.*, 2005). A significant proportion of expenditure in healthcare is used for children, and, with the increased ability to sustain the lives of premature infants, the proportion of spending in child health is likely to rise. This is therefore a major limitation if such calculations are used in estimating cost-effectiveness for national resources.

A further problem with the trade-offs model is that it does not incorporate uncertainty. There is always an element of uncertainty in cost–benefit analysis, as the expected benefits are subject to how a patient's condition progresses or whether health benefits that are expected are forthcoming. In many cases, patients may have multiple pathologies which means that the expected results from a given intervention may be confounded by changes in another aspect of their health. It may also be rendered inaccurate by developments in medicine and technology which mean that a previously untreatable disorder becomes treatable. Thus, trading off can only be done on the premise that diseases progress as expected, without confounding events or changes in scientific knowledge which might alter outcomes. Therefore, these will never be absolute and unchanging.

Arnsen and Norheim (2003) argue that the attempt to quantify quality of life is itself a contradiction in terms as quality and individual perceptions of this in relation to health cannot be reduced to numerical measurements. The 'time trade-off' approach is nevertheless the most widely used method to adjust the quantity of life years for the quality of life years in cost analysis (Arnsen and Norheim, 2003; Griebsch *et al.*, 2005).

THE PLACE OF COST WITHIN HIERARCHIES OF EVIDENCE

The place which cost should hold in hierarchies of evidence is debatable. Unlike other forms of evidence, such as RCTs, there are no hard-and-fast rules regarding how evidence of cost should be rated or regarded. Although how the evidence of cost was gathered should be assessed for any evidence of bias, whether the cost is current or projected, and whether the costs and savings are taken into account, there are no hierarchies of cost in the way that, for example, RCTs hold the highest place in the hierarchy of evidence of positivist inquiry. It cannot be absolutely stated that cost will be more or less important than, for instance, expert opinion. The importance of cost will depend upon the strength of other forms of evidence and the cost in question. NICE have been accused of weighting cost inappropriately in some cases, but claim that cost-effectiveness informs but is not the sole determinant of the institute's guidance (Rawlins *et al.*, 2001). For example, in their recommendations regarding glatiramer acetate and interferon beta for multiple sclerosis, they acknowledged that cost was a major issue, but denied that it was the overriding issue (NICE, 2002g).

ETHICS AND RESOURCE ALLOCATION

The ethical principles which underpin healthcare must be included in the decisions which are made about cost. These principles are beneficence, non-maleficence, justice and autonomy.

The concepts of beneficence and non-maleficence require staff to do good and to do no harm. However, as this chapter has already identified, to do good to one patient may leave inadequate resources for good to be done to another patient. Thus, to simply state that healthcare staff must take the action which will produce most good for one individual patient is too simplistic. At ward level, it may be in the best interests of one patient to have one nurse completely allocated to their care. This may maximise their psychological as well as physical recovery. However, if there are 24 patients on the ward and four nurses, to provide this staff–patient ratio would be detrimental to other patients' well-being. When decisions are made as to which staff will provide care for which patients, the good of each individual patient is effectively weighed up with the needs of all, and decisions made about how the available staff time will be divided between all the patients. Similarly, while it might be beneficial for one patient to have a one-hour outpatient consultation with a consultant physician, this might leave very little time for another 20 patients. Thus, every day, almost unthinkingly, healthcare decisions are made in which the best interests of individual patients are weighed up with the best interests of a larger group. The way in which the nursing workload is allocated at staff handovers, and the decisions about how long a 'slot' each patient in a clinic should have, represent a form of decision-making about rationing in which individual and corporate good are essentially weighed up.

Two ethical positions which may be in conflict in relation to resource allocation are the utilitarian view and one, which judges an action solely on the benefit of its own outcome, isolated from broader consequences. This latter view would maintain that if a treatment were beneficial it should be given. This view would hold that the only consideration of each practitioner should be the patient with whom they are engaged at the time and that doing good and avoiding doing harm to them should be their only concern. If a patient needs care, it should be given, and, if a patient needs to spend an hour with a physician, this should be possible. However, despite the attractiveness of this view, it may be considered incompatible with the complexities of healthcare in which decisions made in relation to one patient will inevitably impact on the resources available for others.

Utilitarian principles are often seen as taking the opposite stance and are used to justify decisions regarding the rationing of healthcare. Utilitarianism requires decisions to be made over what will be the most productive use of resources and the greatest good for the greatest number (Draper and Sorell, 2002). Here, the benefit for individuals is taken in the context of benefit for populations as a whole. This has been linked strongly with the ethical principle of justice.

The principle of justice aims to provide all individuals with equal access to what might be considered a basic need such as health (Wilmot, 2003). However, this is not easy to achieve as it includes local and national resource allocation for a range of health-related conditions (Fletcher and Buka, 1999; Bridges *et al.*, 2001). Although utilitarian principles may be closer to realistically achieving justice in a cost-constrained service than deontological thoughts, given the differing views on what constitutes health and what the priorities within this are, and what is seen as beneficial or harmful, achieving justice in healthcare remains problematic. In addition, utilitarianism may not be seen as entirely just, as what is the best for the greatest number is the dictate, and not what is best for all. It may therefore be seen as unjust by those for whom the best treatment is deemed too costly to be a good use of national resources. The aim of government policy may necessarily be to achieve good health for all population groups and the best care for the greatest number of people, not equal healthcare provision for all individuals (Kazanjian, 2001). This means that treatments which could be the best option for some client groups will not be funded. It also means that the concept of what is deemed to be good health for populations as well as individuals must be identified, which is hugely problematic. However, Norheim (1999) suggests that if such decisions are reached via reliably gathered public opinion this is probably the most acceptable way forward.

The ethical principle of autonomy is currently high on the healthcare agenda. Chapter 9 discusses in detail the concept of patient choice and autonomy, and Chapter 8, professional autonomy. The reality is that, while patient autonomy is the goal, the choices which individuals have in healthcare are real-world choices, and cost is a part of this. An individual's decisions about their holidays may be completely autonomous, in that they can choose where they go, how they get there, how long they stay and what they do while they are there. However, these decisions will still be tempered by reality. If there is no flight from Heathrow to Buenos Aires at midday on a Saturday, you cannot fly there at that time, from that airport, however autonomous you are. Your autonomy means that you will be able to choose what best fits your needs from the available options, for example a flight at 11 a.m. from Heathrow or a flight at midday from Gatwick. Choices must always be in the real world, and cost is a part of this. There is not usually a flight to Buenos Aires every hour because, amongst other things, there is not enough demand to justify the cost of putting these on, and, if there were to be this number of flights, the flights to other destinations would need to be reduced, in order to accommodate them, and cost might be a little higher to compensate for the fact that each plane was half full. This would mean that while those wishing to fly to Buenos Aires would have an excellent service, at high cost, those flying elsewhere would be disadvantaged. Thus, the autonomous traveller must function in a world in which the needs of others must be, and are, also taken into account. The same applies in healthcare.

HOW TO RATION CARE

There is no doubt that some form of rationing of healthcare is inevitable, and decisions must be made as to how resources will be used. Caplan (1992) states that the choices regarding approaches to rationing in healthcare are:

Strict Egalitarianism

Each individual effectively has a voucher for a set amount of healthcare, and, once this has been given, they have no more. Thus, if an infant used all their resources in the first week of life, they would have none left.

Medical Necessity

In this situation, only care which is medically necessary is provided. However, defining medical necessity is problematic and includes the debate on what is reasonable health and for how long life should be sustained, and debate over whether quality or quantity of life is to be valued more, and how quality of life is determined (Scott, 2003).

Adequate Care

Here all individuals should have access to adequate care, but again uncertainty is likely to exist over what is thought to be adequate care. My views of adequate care provision and those of one of my fellow hikers were clarified on a seven-day hike in the Tasmanian bush. Accessing the trail required a flight in a four-seater aircraft to a deserted runway deep in the wilderness. When the weather was bad, flights stopped and our own flight out was deferred for two days for this very reason. In my view, we needed fairly decent first-aid kit, especially because we had two teenagers with us, for whom we had some degree of responsibility. I asked one of the two other adults with whom we would be hiking, the one who was deemed to be the carrier of the first-aid kit, whether he had enough kit. 'I think I've got everything we need,' he replied. I suggested we compare, so as to avoid taking duplicate items. He produced a bottle of tea tree oil and some plasters. My concerns over carrying duplicate kit were unfounded, but it was clear that our ideas of adequate medical care in the bush were different. If we each allocated national health resources based on our idea of adequacy, the outcome would probably also be very different.

Equal Opportunity

This approach means that all individuals have the right to an equal chance to enjoy the range of life's opportunities. Healthcare must be distributed so as to compensate for the disabilities which disease, dysfunction or impairment cause. However, some people have such severe disabilities that full compensation of these would leave no resources for anything else.

Age-based

Allocating resources based on age means that all individuals should have the chance to live a normal life span. This requires a normal life span to be defined, which can be problematic, in some cases frighteningly so for those of us over the age of 30. Three years ago, one of my friends died in a road traffic accident in France. For some reason, I told this to a group of first-year preregistration nursing students. They looked mildly sympathetic that my friend had died, and one of them asked how old she was. '38,' I replied. Their expressions changed slightly. Still sympathetic, but with the clear view that, while it was a shame she had died suddenly, without saying goodbye, at 38, her life was pretty much over anyway. I was four years younger than her. It was a scary thought that, were I to end up in their care, they might casually flick my ventilator's on/off button on the basis that I had had a pretty good innings and might as well quit while I was ahead.

This range of models, and the debate on QALYs, demonstrates that there is no one right way to determine resource allocation justly. Recommendations and guidelines from organisations such as NICE can be seen as one method of reaching the inevitable decisions which must be made about rationing. In this way, they may serve as a tool for improving the quality and consistency of decisions about rationing. It may not mean that decisions are 'right', in part because, as this chapter has outlined, there is no one right way to make such decisions, or any one right decision. However, it will possibly improve the consistency of decision-making and provide a rationale for this. Such decisions can then be viewed as being made on a basis of equality of provision across the country and between specialities, rather than potentially inconsistent decisions being made by individual practitioners dependent on their personal value or beliefs. In this way, they may serve as a tool for improving the quality and consistency of decisions about rationing. It may also reduce the potential for blame to be attributed to individual practitioners by patients for the finite nature of healthcare funding and the reality that not all treatment or care options can be provided, or provided within the timeframe that they would like. Clinical guidelines and care protocols may thus offer some degree of protection for staff as they can identify to patients what will and what will not be funded, and why this is. However, it does mean that limits on patient choices and practitioner's range of care options are likely to exist.

Clinical guidelines and care protocols will not remove the issue of cost in healthcare. In many ways, they will highlight it by making explicit what will and what will not be funded.

SUMMARY

Evidence-based practice, of which clinical guidelines and care protocols form a part, is intended to be real-world practice, and thus cost, which is a part of the real world of healthcare, is a part of clinical guidelines and care protocols. There is no intention for the guidance developed at a national level to be divorced from the reality of cost. The reality of cost in a national health service which is free at the point of delivery means that there is not infinite funding for the infinite and ever-increasing demand for healthcare. The intention of guidance such as that issued by NICE is to achieve a balance between clinical efficacy and cost-effectiveness and improve the equity of care provision. However, it will not enable absolute and unlimited choice for staff or patients. Nevertheless, whilst accepting that not all treatment or care can be funded, and that difficult decisions will have to be made concerning resources, healthcare staff and the public should be involved in debating what constitutes the best use of resources.

Although national guidance is seen as one method of standardising what care provision is available and providing greater equity across populations, there is also a cost to developing such guidance, and this must also be taken from central resources (Hughes, 2002). Chapter 5 identified that the process of guideline development is potentially time-consuming and costly, and the implementation of guidelines may take considerable time and effort. The costs involved in this process must therefore also be weighed in the balance of improving the cost-effectiveness of healthcare by the use of clinical guidelines. Keaney and Lorimer (1999) identify that developing national guidelines represents a significant investment of NHS resources, and question whether the investment is recouped from improvements in practice once guidelines are developed. If the cost of developing a guideline is excessive and the potential benefit small, or only likely to assist a small proportion of the population, the cost may not be justifiable. One problem is that without undertaking the guideline development process it will not be possible to say whether cost benefit will be considerable or borderline. However, one of the criteria by which NICE select or do not select subjects for guideline development is whether a significant percentage of the population will be assisted by it.

Given the complexity of defining what constitutes quality of life and health, it will also not be easy to give guidance which adequately balances clinical efficacy and cost-effectiveness. There are no gold standard tools to measure cost-effectiveness in healthcare, and although incremental cost-effectiveness ratios and trade-off models such as QALYs are often used, these approaches have flaws.

There is no easy answer to how healthcare resources should be allocated, but one thing which is clear is that cost is a real issue in healthcare, and in the development and use of clinical guidelines and care protocols.

11
Politics, Power, Guidelines and Protocols

This chapter discusses the political agendas involved in the popularisation and use of clinical guidelines and care protocols. In Chapter 1 some of the political drivers behind the move towards using clinical guidelines and care protocols were suggested. Other chapters have debated the implications which clinical guidelines and care protocols have for professional freedom and autonomy, patient choices in healthcare and the place of cost in healthcare. These all occur in the context of a health service which is publicly funded. The governing political party's responsibility for healthcare provision includes ensuring that public money is well spent, and, if they wish to remain in office, they must demonstrate a commitment to providing equal standards of high-quality, cost-effective healthcare to all. As clinical guidelines and care protocols are linked to these goals, the government, principally via the DoH, are likely to have an influence in how national guidelines and protocols are developed and used. For similar reasons of demonstrating a commitment to quality, equality and cost-effectiveness, local political influences, at the levels of local government and Trust government, will affect the development and use of local clinical guidelines and care protocols.

Although political influences have been alluded to in previous chapters, this chapter focuses on the political aspects of clinical guidelines and care protocols. It discusses the events which have resulted in the development of national clinical guidelines and the aim to develop standardised national care protocols from a political perspective. It then considers the relationship between politicians and healthcare staff, the relationships between healthcare staff groups and how these affect and are affected by the drive towards using clinical guidelines and care protocols.

DEMONSTRATING QUALITY

Chapter 1 identified that concerns over standards of healthcare provision have contributed to the current drive towards evidence-based practice. Politically, healthcare is a major election issue. Thus, demonstrating that achieving quality healthcare is a priority is important for all political parties, and demonstrating the provision of good-quality healthcare and that any perceived shortfalls have been addressed is important for the existing government.

The notion of developing national clinical guidelines and care protocols has been supported by the Labour government, with the stated aim of these documents improving the quality and consistency of care provision. Clinical guidelines and care protocols also have the unstated but nonetheless clear aim of reassuring the public that the government are committed to addressing some identified deficits in the quality and equity of healthcare provision. The evolution of NICE and the associated development of national clinical guidelines was strongly related to the recommendations from the Bristol Inquiry (Kennedy, 2001). One of the rationales for their development was to assure the public that there will be an increasing number of defined standards of healthcare provision which they can expect will be adhered to. Inquiries such as that which followed the events in paediatric cardiac surgery at Bristol are conducted independently of government. The governing political party must nonetheless be seen to support the measures recommended by such investigations so as to demonstrate a commitment to quality of care and to an effective use of public money. Thus, following the events of Bristol and the recommendations arising from the Bristol Inquiry, the DoH have openly promoted the development and use of national guidance related to certain aspects of healthcare.

Clinical guidelines and care protocols form two of the four principal methods which the DoH (2003) suggest for maintaining, improving and monitoring quality in healthcare. The other two are quality-assurance systems and standards, both of which can be associated with clinical guidelines or care protocols. Clinical guidelines and care protocols may be considered to outline the standards of care and methods of care provision which are expected of individuals and organisations. They may also be used to measure whether or not the recommended steps in care provision have been adhered to or the aims of guidelines or protocols achieved. Thus, clinical guidelines and care protocols may become a part of clinical standards and quality-assurance systems, and they therefore play a central part in the government's recommendations for achieving and demonstrating the provision of quality of care.

However, as has been highlighted in previous chapters, there is no absolute consensus on what constitutes quality care, and the measurement of quality of care using any method is not fail-safe. It is almost impossible to accurately assess all aspects of the quality of healthcare provision. The fact that clinical guidelines or care protocols have been followed does not necessarily mean that all aspects of care provision have been of high quality, or that patients believe that they have received quality care (Warne and McAndrew, 2004; Long, 2003). Although good guidelines make recommendations based on the current best evidence, there is no guarantee that all clinical guidelines or care protocols are of high quality. Using well-developed clinical guidelines or care protocols which are based on good evidence as a quality indicator can show whether a specific aspect of care was provided at a standard commensurate with what has been decided is acceptable quality. However, they do not, and cannot, and neither are they intended to, measure the entire care experience. Nevertheless, they mean that a statement can be made by those who must account for healthcare as to whether or not certain aspects of care have been planned and delivered in accordance with what is deemed to be best practice.

Clinical guidelines and care protocols are not only endorsed by central government but also form a part of government targets for the achievement of quality. There is, therefore, as discussed in Chapter 8, some pressure exerted for individuals and NHS Trusts to use national clinical guidelines and to develop and use care protocols. In some instances, financial penalties exist for any non-attainment of the standards laid down in clinical guidelines (DoH, 2002) and the existence of care protocols related to some areas of practice is a factor which is assessed in determining the star ratings of NHS Trusts (NHS Modernisation Agency and NICE, 2004a). Adherence to national clinical guidelines and the creation of care protocols thus have implications for the funding of NHS Acute Trusts and Primary Care Trusts, the autonomy of Trust management and the ongoing employment of managers. If a government is seen to take action against those who fail to achieve set standards, some of which are linked to clinical guidelines and care protocols, then they can claim that they are taking steps to ensure the provision of quality care, and acting upon problems in achieving the prescribed standard of care. However, this introduces a significant element of duress on individuals and organisations to develop or use, and be seen to use, clinical guidelines and care protocols. As was suggested in Chapter 8, high-profile quality problems which the NHS have encountered mean that it may be justifiable for the activities of healthcare staff to be more tightly controlled and for them to have less autonomy. However, how far a decrease in autonomy created by the implementation of national standards will actually influence the quality of patient care for the better is debatable.

NICE AND POLITICAL INFLUENCES

National clinical guidelines for England and Wales are developed by NICE, as recommended in the Kennedy Report (2001). NICE are independent of government in relation to party politics, but they are advised by government ministers on what can be justified as a use of NHS resources. The decision regarding what subjects will be covered in clinical guidelines is also strongly influenced by government ministers and thus the priorities of the dominant political party inevitably influence the areas in which national guidance is developed. This may be appropriate, so that funding is streamlined and used most effectively to target major national health issues which affect a significant proportion of the population and to ensure cohesion between health-related spending. However, it also means that, although the actual guidance issued by NICE, for example whether or not an intervention can be recommended for use, should be free of party-political influence, the guideline development process is inevitably influenced by government.

That cost is a real consideration in healthcare has been a consistent theme in this book. Thus, in the politics of healthcare, cost is likely to be a significant issue. As well as reassuring the public that they are doing their utmost to ensure high standards of care, governments must also demonstrate that they are using the taxpayers' money responsibly. For politicians, as well as the need to demonstrate that quality care has been achieved, there is therefore a need to demonstrate that healthcare-related spending has been appropriate and effective. NICE are considered to be independent of government; however, their creation, funding and continued existence largely depend on funding from the DoH. Thus, it is reasonable to assume that they, like other areas of the NHS, must be able to demonstrate that they are cost-effective and that the advice which they give contributes to cost-effective care provision as well as clinically effective care.

Equally, there is the potential, if not an actual, problem that NICE may recommend care or treatment which would produce a high standard of healthcare without the necessary resources to enable Trusts to achieve this being made available. Although the resources available for healthcare are finite, and the demand infinite, where new treatment is recommended which is more costly than existing treatment, how Trusts will be able to provide this without being given additional funding is not always evident. Although this may appear to be an oversight in the planning of national guidance, it is possible that it will give the impression that governments are enabling NICE to recommend better treatment, and thus are, by proxy, promoting high-quality care. It is then seen as the responsibility of individual professionals or organisations to provide this standard of care, and they, not the government, are seen as responsible for any shortfall. Politically, this may seem a good tactic, but it will not do anything to improve actual patient care.

EXPANDED ROLES AND PROTOCOLS

One function of care protocols is intended to be to assist in the expansion of the roles that can be undertaken by healthcare staff and thus to facilitate more expedient use of the available skills. The *NHS Plan* (DoH, 2000) states that the government intend that care-protocol use will allow the expansion of the scope of tasks which nurses and other professions allied to medicine are permitted to carry out. The DoH consider that this will enable healthcare professionals to fulfil roles that make the best use of their knowledge and competence, and which will most effectively meet patients' needs rather than roles being restricted in accordance with an individual's professional identity. The DoH (2000) claim that enabling nursing staff, and other professions allied to medicine, to undertake a wider range of roles will result in the reduction of waiting times, improve the continuity of care for individuals and make more effective and efficient use of resources. The potential expansion of healthcare roles in association with care protocol use has a number of implications for professions and patients, which will be discussed later in the chapter. However, the political agendas involved appear to include taking visible steps to improve the quality of care, for example by improved continuity of care, improved communication and reduction of cost. They may also serve the government's purpose of wooing professions allied to medicine with suggestions of a greater valuing of their performance. Being valued is not always a vastly positive thing. Most restaurants claim to value their customers, but this is probably because their customers are what pays their bills, not because they like their customers, or the way they eat. They are getting an income and the customers' value relates to this. Supermarkets give 'great value offers' of two items for the price of one. When I am told that my contribution is valued, I am always filled with dismay, because it usually means that I am about to be asked to do something for nothing and to see the fact that I am valued as enough reward. This has been illustrated in both practice and education settings in the recent past.

After a bout of travelling, I decided to play a little financial catch-up by doing a few shifts on a local paediatric unit, as an agency nurse. One memorable afternoon, the nurse manager confided in me that because she 'valued me' I was to join the nurse bank, instead of the agency. This would result in me receiving £14.50 an hour on a Sunday instead of the £51.50 that the agency paid me. When I asked what the other benefits would be, I received a glare and the tale of my great value was reiterated. I have no delusions about the value of my skills and knowledge: I can get a nappy in the right place two out of three times and do a few bits of other low-key stuff, but nothing really spectacular. However, the idea that she felt that she valued me so much that she would like to pay me £37 an hour less than I was getting was interesting. The issue of cost and rationing of resources, including the resources for staff pay in healthcare is, of course, complex. Had she said that she couldn't afford to pay the agency rates because if she did all her money would be gone in one day and the children would be left without nurses for the rest of the year, I might have been sympathetic. Had she said that she needed something cheap and nasty and I had all the necessary qualities, I might have been mildly insulted. However, her belief that the 'you are valued' story was one I would fall for when I was being invited to lose £444 for a 12-hour shift was even more insulting.

From an educational slant, it has been perhaps even more bizarre. I was asked if I would care to give a lecture on something or other at a university near me and was offered £20 per hour. I felt this to be a tad ungenerous, as I was a senior lecturer, with a doctorate, and this was my specialist subject. When I questioned this, using the listed payscales as my argument, I was told that consultants would be paid £45, SpRs £35 and nurses £20, but that they wanted a nurse as they valued the nursing side of the subject being the focus – so much that they would pay me £25 hour less than a medical consultant, who would not provide the focus which was so valued.

I leave you to surmise what I did.

This is, of course, the cynical view, but it is worth being aware of. It may mean nurses are cheap at the price, or that they provide a cost-effective solution, not that the government value the concept and philosophy of expert holistic nursing. This move may therefore improve patient care, be more cost-effective and improve job satisfaction for some staff, but other potential political dimensions should not be ignored.

The development of national clinical guidelines and the suggestion that national care protocols should be developed therefore has a significant political agenda in terms of a government demonstrating that quality care in the NHS is being addressed, and in achieving or appearing to achieve cost-effectiveness. Although ostensibly the professions and government both have the aim of enhancing patient care, the precise intentions of each party are not necessarily the same, and, as well as the precise focus of each party's intentions, power dynamics between government and professions influence and are influenced by the moves to using clinical guidelines and care protocols.

CHANGES IN THE ORGANISATION OF HEALTHCARE

Differences of opinion and issues over the balance of power between healthcare staff and government are not new. Medical staff and politicians have rarely, since the inception of the NHS, found easy ways of agreeing about its existence, what it should provide and how it should be managed (Winyard, 2003). Although the NHS is publicly funded, and thus ultimately administered by government ministers, healthcare professions, by their existence and managerial functions within it, are intended to form a part of the balance against undue party-political influence in the NHS. However, healthcare staff, and within this each profession, are not a homogeneous group. The way in which a politician and a surgeon view cost may differ. The way in which a physician and a nurse view cost may also differ, as may the way in which a consultant who is a head of directorate and a junior doctor see cost. The way in which a ward manager who is responsible for their budget sees cost may differ from how an SHO sees cost. Thus, although this section appears to discuss politics as if it were a simple split between politicians and healthcare professionals, and between professional groups, the reality is that healthcare professions are composed of a number of different professions, and of different managerial levels and individuals within these professions, all of whom may see political issues differently. The same applies to an extent to politicians. Thus, any discussion of politics in healthcare is necessarily a generalisation to what seems to be the dominant view of each group. The debates in this chapter relate to the politics of government and healthcare professionals as a whole, and to the politics between healthcare groups as a whole. This comes with the caveat that this type of debate inevitably simplifies the complex structures of government and healthcare professionals.

The power relationship between government and healthcare professionals and between different healthcare professionals will dictate how far each party's view influences decisions regarding healthcare provision and the use of healthcare resources. Later on in the chapter, the power differentials between various members of the healthcare professons will be discussed in more detail. However, although a number of professional groups make up the multidisciplinary team which provides healthcare, the focus of relationships between politicians and healthcare professionals tends to be on that between medicine and politicians.

Historically, it has been medical staff who have been predominantly involved in debates on policy and politics, with the initial development of the NHS significantly influenced by the power which medical staff held (Wilmot, 2003). To a great degree, this situation, in which medical staff are the principal power players, persists, although the power which medicine has traditionally wielded appears to be faltering in relation to government. The NHS was created on the basis that it would be a hospital-dominated system for delivering medical care, meaning that its main focus was medicine, with the consultants who ran hospitals controlling the majority of NHS resources. It was initially medical staff who were in charge of hospitals and thus had responsibility for financial decisions, bed availability and overall service management. Medical staff allegedly became the leaders of healthcare and managers of hospitals because of the philosophy of hospitals being set up to treat physical ill health. They were the individuals to whom patients presented themselves, they decided whether or not an individual was ill and, because of their subsequent role in diagnosing disease, referring on and coordinating care, theirs was the central focus of healthcare provision. There is a suggestion that medical staff have been the dominant party in healthcare politics, not because of their scientific knowledge or the success of medical interventions but because of their political acumen in ensuring that they have retained a central control of the NHS (Wilmot, 2003).

Although healthcare is provided by a range of professionals, the politics of healthcare and control and power therein often allude to the power differential between medicine and nursing. The fact that, historically, medical doctors were men and nurses were women, in a society in which women were seen as politically naive and subordinate to men, probably contributed to the dominance which medicine enjoyed (Wilmot, 2003). The fact that a part of nurses' role in providing care for patients has been perceived as being to carry out the instructions of medical staff has been built upon this power equation (Hewitt, 2002). The expanding roles which nurses have taken on, and the changing gender demographics of medical school entrants, might be expected to alter this, but they have not apparently significantly affected the power relationship between medicine and nursing (Martin, 1998; Wilmot, 2003).

The position of hospital-based medicine in relation to resource management has been altered by reorganisations of the NHS. Responsibility for hospital management has shifted from medical staff to general managers. Medical staff are thus no longer usually in charge of hospitals, although medical directors tend to manage a great deal of the business of hospital directorates. There has also been a shift towards community-based care, health promotion and public health, rather than hospital-based care aimed at curing ill health. This means that medically dominated tertiary-care centres no longer necessarily hold the balance of power or financial resources.

PROFESSIONAL AUTONOMY

Although hospitals are no longer necessarily managed by healthcare professionals, professions have, as identified in Chapter 8, enjoyed and expect to continue to hold a significant degree of autonomy in their structure and function (Wilmot, 2003). Medical staff have, for many years, enjoyed relative freedom from political influence, and have been largely self-governed and autonomous. However, well-publicised cases of medical misconduct such as the Shipman Inquiry (Smith, 2005) have brought into question medicine's ability to self-govern. The subject of medical regulation, and how this should be managed so as to ensure that the public are protected, has therefore become politicised and appears to aim to make medicine more publicly accountable (Salter, 2001).

The debates which have ensued over the calls for changes to medical regulation have some parallels to the arguments surrounding clinical guidelines and care protocols. It has been argued that the Health Act 1999 and associated government policies are bringing about a shift from medicine being self-regulated to regulation being government-driven and interventionist. Although changes to medical regulation have the espoused aim of protecting the public, in the same way that the use of national guidance has the espoused aim of maximising the quality of care, it has been suggested that the reason for the change is also strongly associated with a concern with cost (Davies, 2000). Although medical regulation itself does not directly affect the cost of care, if government influence over medicine is increased, they may be better able to control the activities of medical staff and thus exert greater control over the cost of care provision (Davies, 2000). Politically, however, it will appear more attractive to the public that politicians are seeking to control medical staff to protect patients than to control costs. There is also the obvious conclusion to be drawn that this will be an opportunity for government to reduce medical power and thus for politicians to have greater control of healthcare.

The changes in management of the NHS over the years and recent moves to alter medical regulation therefore have the potential to alter the power which medicine holds in relation to overall healthcare provision. They also have the potential to influence the power which medicine holds relative to other healthcare professions.

POWER BETWEEN PROFESSIONS

Although political debates have usually focused on the relationship between medicine and politicians, nurses are the largest group of employees in the NHS. They should, therefore, perhaps logically wield a significant degree of power (Macdonald and Bodzak, 1999). However, Antrobus and Kitson (1999) suggest that health policy has, to date, been developed with limited input from nursing. As nurses are the professional group who arguably spend the most time with each individual patient, it could be argued that their understanding of the patient's perspective will be the most accurate and that their input is therefore important in influencing policy. However, although the nature of nursing work predisposes nurses to being perhaps best placed to represent their patients' interests, it has been suggested that the nature of nursing work has also been one of nursing's difficulties in achieving political power over the years. This situation may now be changing as a result of alterations in the roles which nurses and medical staff take on and nurses being increasingly independent in their practice. The power of the medical profession is said, at least in part, to stem from the fact that doctors were responsible for diagnosing and defining a patient's health needs and acting as the first point of contact and referral point (Blank and Burau, 2004). This pattern may now be altering. The DoH suggest that, with the use of care protocols, it will be possible for nurses to manage entire caseloads and, possibly, to be the point of referral to other agencies and professions.

Although some medical staff have welcomed this move, and there have been reports of positive outcomes, for example of surgical assistant roles (Kneebone and Darzi, 2005), there has been some concern over it within some professional contexts. On medicine's part, the stated concern is usually whether nurses will be able to manage the complexity of such roles, or have the knowledge or skills required. Thus, ostensibly, patient safety is their concern. However, although patient safety is the usual stated concern, it must also be postulated that the possible decline in medical power which this will bring must be a consideration. This has been to some extent evident in the concerns expressed by surgeons regarding the employment of surgical assistants. The debate over the employment of surgical assistants has followed the usual pattern of debates on extending roles and employing new groups of staff to undertake medical or surgical tasks. Ability to perform discrete tasks is usually able to be assured, but whether practitioners will have the breadth of knowledge needed to manage entire patient situations, including complications or unexpected outcomes, is the focus of debate. This is clearly related to patient safety. However, this has been accompanied by concerns over how junior surgical staff will learn if surgical assistants take on many minor surgical roles. The logical argument is that surgical trainees can learn a great deal from a variety of healthcare workers, including nurses, physiotherapists, occupational therapists, assistant grades from various professional backgrounds and ward domestic staff. Whether surgical house officers and registrars are prepared to do this may be a comment on their professional territorialism rather than the skills and knowledge of other staff and their ability to teach them.

Other medical staff may welcome the move to allow other professions or assistants to work with them and adopt some of their roles. However, whether they in fact value the contribution which others make to care, and the skills and knowledge that they bring, is open to debate. In some cases, they may indeed value the knowledge and skills which nurses and other professionals have, respect them, and believe that them taking on additional roles enhances care provision. A distinction should nonetheless be made between valuing individuals or groups in this way and welcoming a group or individual who is willing to take on some aspects of one's work and thus reduce one's workload. Valuing the contribution of another individual or group is different from being glad that someone else is willing to take on some of one's work.

Understanding why nursing has remained subordinate to medicine, despite nurses being the largest group of NHS employees, merits consideration. Academically, many nurses now hold degree-level and above qualifications and thus are academically equally well qualified as doctors, and in a rising number of cases hold superior academic qualifications to medical staff, albeit in a different discipline. Despite being the most consistent and central theme in defining nursing (McCance *et al.*, 1999), and its almost undisputed central function (Henderson, 1966; Watson, 1985; Leninger, 1991), the interpretation of the word 'care' has possibly contributed to nursings' failure to achieve political power. Caring has sometimes been linked with the view of nurses as nurturing (Scott, 2003), with an apolitical concern for individual patients, compared with a view of medical staff focusing on scientific decision-making regarding interventions aimed at cure, imposing technical-rational decisions on nurses and patients alike without engagement in interpersonal aspects of patient care

(Hewitt, 2002; Scott, 2003). In addition, the culture in which medicine thrived was one in which medical paternalism was seen as acceptable, where making decisions on behalf of others, regarding their health and even continuation of life, was seen as part of a doctor's duty. Such paternalism inevitably brings with it power, to make decisions for others, and while this inevitably involves responsibility, in the case of decisions about life and death perhaps an unenviable responsibility, that responsibility brings with it power.

Interestingly, medical staff are now being encouraged to become more 'caring'. This includes them engaging in discussions with patients, promoting openness and honesty and power sharing with patients, understanding the holistic nature of illness and desisting from their traditional paternalistic stance and their detachment from patients. If medicine rose to power because of the tendency for medical staff to impose decisions on patients and other staff, the changes in the view of medical paternalism bring with them changes in the power which medicine can yield.

This, and the changing roles of professions, may mean that medicine becomes less dominant, as its stance and that of nursing become closer. This may result in the professions jointly retaining power in healthcare and the distribution of that power being more equal. However, while this may seem attractive to many parties, particularly to nursing and professions allied to medicine, this change may not in fact enable other professions, or even the public, to increase their power; it may simply mean that governments become more dominant in healthcare decision-making and healthcare professionals collectively lose power. Power shifting from one profession may, therefore, not enhance the power of another. The balance may simply move out of healthcare and, despite assurances to the contrary, may not move to patients.

THE NATURE OF POWER

Power is not something which can be easily moved from one group or one individual to another (Canter, 2001). It is also unlikely that any individual or group with significant power will be easily convinced to yield this to another (Freire, 1970). Thus, it is realistic to expect that medicine will be unwilling to allow government to reduce its power or that it will willingly share power with other professions or patients.

The ability of government to reduce the power of medicine is relatively strong, particularly following cases such as Bristol and Shipman. However, unsurprisingly, it appears unlikely that medicine will easily accept a reduction in power. There is a potential for attempts to redress the balance of power between medicine and government to involve other parties, notably nursing, professions allied to medicine and the public. The reduction in medical power which any government seeks may appear to give more power to other professions such as nursing, or patients. However, those apparently benefiting from this shift should be certain that it is a move which genuinely empowers them, not covert control from another party or by another means. Like oppressive regimes which give the impression of valuing those they oppress in an attempt to continue their subordination (Freire, 1970), medicine may apparently value nursing and allied professions, or patients' views. In reality, they may wish to continue their subordination while making them allies against the common foe of government. Government may wish to gain favour with nursing or patients so as to gain allies against medicine, and to weaken overall healthcare power and strengthen their own position, not to increase the power of other professions or patients. They may also see this as a way to reduce costs if, for example, nurses are cheaper to employ than medical staff. Thus, those apparently benefiting from changes in power demographics should be aware of the possible reasons for the opportunities which they are offered. This is not to say that these should not be taken, but that they should be taken in an informed manner.

As well as the many tactics which a dominant group may use to retain power, those seeking redress of power must want this, and see themselves as in need of it (Freire, 1970). Nursing and other allied professions must, in order to gain greater power, want this and actively seek to change the power dynamic. It cannot be assumed that the fault for nursing's lack of political power lies outside nursing. Nurses may not wish to challenge their political place or may not see this as a priority. Maslin-Prothero *et al.* (2002) suggest that many nurses in the United Kingdom accept the model which places them outside the political power domain, regarding politics as an undesirable distraction from their core purpose of care delivery. Thus, nurses may not themselves truly oppose the medically dominant scheme of power, or the power of government, or wish to increase their own involvement in national and local decision-making. That is the profession's choice, but, if this is a choice that nursing collectively makes, by decision or default, then it is responsible for this.

CHANGING ROLES

The suggestion that using care protocols can increase the role remit of professions allied to medicine may be an example of where mixed motives for apparently valuing the skills and knowledge of professions allied to medicine exist. The DoH (2000) see care-protocol use as expanding the scope of nursing practice, and valuing the skills and knowledge which nurses have. This includes nurses prescribing drugs, treating patients with minor injuries in accident and emergency departments and taking the lead role in managing patient caseloads (DoH, 2000). Riley and Peters (2000) suggest that widening the role of the nurse is also one of the best ways of improving the cost-effectiveness and quality of patient care. In this respect, the DoH's (2000) stance may therefore be seen as likely to improve care provision and the efficiency of use of resources as well as publicly demonstrating that they value nurses.

The expansion of the role of the nurse is not a new concept. The Department of Health and Social Security (1977) recognised this idea and defined such role expansion as nurses performing activities not catered for in basic nurse training. This generally focused on the acquisition of the skills which enable nurses to perform tasks traditionally carried out by medical staff (Cole and Shanley, 1998). The Scope of Professional Practice (UKCC, 1992) developed the concept of the expanded role of the nurse from nurses taking on medical tasks to enlarging the nursing care elements of their role (Cole and Shanley, 1998). However, there is still a tendency for nurses' role development to mean that they take on areas of practice previously carried out by other professional groups, notably medical staff (Jones and Davies, 1999; Riley and Peters, 2000). This may be beneficial for nurses if it represents a move to greater autonomy and decision-making, where they act as the interdisciplinary coordinators of care, referring patients to other agencies or individuals as appropriate, carrying out some investigations and prescribing (DoH, 2000; Kerrins, 2001). However, Riley and Peters (2000) have identified that there is a potential for nurses' role expansion to be reduced to taking on additional skills, tasks or administrative functions from another profession, often medicine, which do little to develop their specialist input into the nursing care of individual patients. Indeed, the suggestion that an expansion of nurses' roles may be achieved by the following of a variety of protocols may mean that nursing expertise is not what is valued. As was discussed in Chapter 8, expertise in care is much more than the ability to follow guidelines or protocols. It involves weighing up the multiple factors which impact on each individual care situation, including making decisions about when the information from clinical guidelines or care protocols should be adhered to and when these should be disregarded.

Thus, having a greater range of options for care provision may allow nurses to provide more holistic care, for example in managing patient caseloads, within which they address all aspects of the individual client's physical, psychological and social needs (DoH, 2000). However, whether an individual is simply performing more tasks for an individual patient or being able to spend a greater amount of time with a patient in a manner which allows them to address their physical, social, psychological, spiritual, intellectual and emotional needs (Rawlins *et al.*, 1993) is the key issue.

The DoH (2000) and RCN (2000) identify that nurses expanding their role will free up medical staff time. Cost-effective solutions to meet the targets for the reduction of junior doctors' hours, address the difficulty in recruiting to some medical specialities and to improve the supervision of doctors in postregistration training must be sought. However, whether nurses taking on these roles is the most appropriate solution is debatable. Whether each element of role expansion is an appropriate or optimum use of nursing time, skill and knowledge and how taking on additional roles will impact on other aspects of patient care traditionally performed by nurses must be considered (Cole and Shanley, 1998) and how they contribute to other professions and overall patient care. There is a risk that, far from valuing nurses, the government are aiming to save money and resolve the problems associated with the reduction of junior doctors' hours. Their intention to give the impression of valuing nursing is likely to be aimed at encouraging nurses to follow this path. They may indeed value nurses, as a ready-made cost-effective solution to many of their problems. However, they may not value the concept of expert holistic nursing care. Politicians may also seek to convince nursing that it is valued, in order to gain allies in healthcare, not because of truly valuing nursing. At the same time, although some medical staff oppose any expansion of nursing roles, it may be that some of those who apparently support the move see it as a method of discarding the less attractive aspects of their roles and simultaneously resolving the problems of covering for reduced junior doctors' hours. They too may suggest that they value nursing, with similar agendas to those of politicians.

While this does not mean that nursing, and other professions allied to medicine, should fail to avail itself of the opportunities that it has and expand and develop its remit, it should be aware of the possible reasons for other professions or politicians apparently valuing nursing. An awareness of these will go some way towards ensuring that nursing and patients, not medicine and politicians, benefit from nursing's skills and knowledge. Using care protocols may be a useful adjunct to nurses developing their roles, but they will only be useful if the focus of role development remains on nursing. The RCN (2005) suggest that in most cases nurses feel that their professionalism and autonomy has been enhanced by expanding their roles, and if this continues this is positive and good. However, the enhancement of nursing practice and patient care, not covert moves to give greater power to government or medicine, should be nursing's aim.

SUMMARY

It is neither possible nor desirable to ignore the political influences which exist in healthcare. In a publicly funded health service, politicians must be able to account for how they use healthcare resources, and thus it is inevitable that a part of a government's agenda will be to show that high-quality care is being provided. Improvements in patient care are the stated reason for the development of clinical guidelines and care protocols, but a significant impetus for their development is also political, to demonstrate a commitment to high-quality care and the achievement of cost-effectiveness.

At the same time, the relative power differential which has existed between healthcare (notably medicine) and government is now being challenged. The changes in power dynamics between government and medicine as well as changes in society and access to information mean that medical paternalism is no longer acceptable. This may affect the power relationships between medicine and society and within the professions. It may result in other professions having greater power. However, it may simply erode the power of medicine without bringing about a change in the power which other professions or patients enjoy.

The suggestion that care protocols may be used to enable professions to widen their remit is a point which merits consideration. This may well be advantageous, and there is evidence that nurses feel that the expansion of their roles allows them to focus on and enhance nursing care, not medical or technical care. However, there is a risk that such expansion being based on care protocols or clinical guidelines will reduce care to a series of technical tasks rather than place the emphasis on holism, which is alleged to be the impetus for expanding roles. There is also the potential for governments and other professions, such as medicine, appearing to value nursing when in fact they are seeking to use this as a part of reorganising the power differentials that exist in their own favour. This should not detract from individuals or professions expanding their role remit, but professions will be well placed to be aware of all the agendas involved in such decisions.

Likewise, clinical guidelines may appear to give greater information to patients and improve care standards by identifying what can be expected. However, there is a risk that these will mean that the cheapest available option, not the most clinically effective, is recommended. It may also mean that, where there are financial or managerial implications for healthcare providers, if targets linked to guidelines or protocols are not met, patient choice is significantly reduced and a degree of coercion used to encourage them to choose to comply with guidelines or protocols. This may include the uptake of screening or the acceptance of treatment or care options which they would not in fact prefer. Thus, rather than patients' power being increased, the power of politicians may be increased and decisions changed from being medically to being politically led.

Although political influences on healthcare may be seen as unsavoury, they, like cost, are a reality of healthcare. Healthcare professionals practise in an environment in which party politics and inter- and intraprofessional politics play a significant role. To be unaware of them is therefore unwise, as they influence everyday practice and the care which can be offered to patients. Medicine has traditionally held the dominant power in healthcare, and this is often commented upon as if the responsibility for this lies with medicine alone. However, this is not the case. If other professions truly oppose the status quo and see altering this as a priority, it is their responsibility to increase their own political involvement so as to alter this. Similarly, with government, it is not enough for healthcare professionals to complain of undue government or political influence. If a profession, or professions, genuinely wishes to change its relative power status, it must be prepared to engage in the necessary political discussions and activity to achieve this. This will require concerted effort and intraprofessional unity, but it is not really sufficient for medical staff, nurses or any other profession to adopt a position of helplessness in relation to government or other professions.

12

Best Practice: Where Do We Go from Here?

The preceding chapters have explored some of the issues involved in developing and using clinical guidelines and care protocols. This includes how clinical guidelines and care protocols fit, or do not fit, with the concept of evidence-based practice, how they can be developed and evaluated, how individuals and organisations can decide whether or not to use existing guidance and how this can be implemented. They have also discussed the financial and professional implications of using clinical guidelines and care protocols, the impact on patient involvement in care and choice and the political issues involved in their popularisation.

The intention of this last chapter is to tie these themes together and to discuss the 'So what?' factor. It aims to discuss how, given all the sometimes conflicting advice and themes which emerge, clinical guidelines and care protocols can be used while simultaneously achieving best practice. The overriding aim of evidence-based practice is that it should be real-world practice, and this means practising in an imperfect world in which there are constraints on care provision, but where the best possible practice within these should be the aim. Best practice is best practice in the real world, not in an unlikely utopia.

Best practice is practice which addresses the specific needs of individual patients, and therefore no text can ever absolutely say what best practice is, because this will always be situation-specific. However, the intention of this chapter is to summarise how clinical guidelines and care protocols can be used in the quest for what form the principles of best practice.

HOW GUIDELINES CAN BEST INFLUENCE PATIENT CARE

Clinical guidelines and care protocols should not be used in isolation, or in all situations. There will be situations in which they should be rejected as inappropriate to the needs of individuals. They should be used to inform health-care staff by providing guidance on what is thought to be the best option regarding a specific aspect of care or the consensus on how a given situation is usually best tackled. They should be used to assist in decision-making and to guide practice. But they cannot and should not be used in an attempt to replace expert decision-making which weighs up all the aspects of each individual situation. Being inanimate, theoretically developed statements, clinical guidelines or care protocols cannot take into account the multiple variables of patient circumstances. They should be seen and used as a part of the wide range of information that informs each practice encounter. They provide guidance but cannot dictate what should be done in every case. Legally and professionally, practitioners are responsible and therefore also accountable for their actions, and, while they can and should use existing guidelines or protocols to assist them in decision-making, they must still be able to say why they did or did not use these in specific cases.

The value of clinical guidelines and care protocols is in their provision of easily accessible information, based on a summary of the current best evidence, on what the most effective approach is likely to be in a 'standard patient'. Given that in the real world there is no such thing as a standard patient, practitioners must then interpret and apply this information to their own practice, where they care for real, non-standard, human beings.

Despite the increasing range of guidelines and protocols, best, or even acceptable, practice is not following a series of guidelines or protocols. Even where a number of protocols or guidelines, or one single guideline, provide input relevant to many aspects of the care of an individual patient, this cannot constitute their whole care. Although clinical guidelines and care protocols can direct or inform on aspects of care provision, the quality of care for individual patients is dictated to a great extent by the personal encounters which link the many aspects of their care. This includes the order in which aspects of care are provided, the communication processes which are involved in care encounters, the manner in which care is provided, tone of voice, touch and empathy. These cannot be prescribed or outlined in guidelines or protocols, but contribute significantly to how patients perceive the quality of their care. They are also likely to affect the outcome of care physically, socially, psychologically and emotionally and patients' inclination to access further healthcare input and therefore their ongoing health.

Most practitioners have always worked in situations where some form of guidelines and protocols exist, and thus their existence is not new. However, with their development at a national level, and the political agendas involved, the issue of the weight that they carry has become more pronounced. In a cost-conscious health service, expert healthcare staff may need to defend the importance of their expertise and how this, rather than simply following guidelines or protocols, produces best practice.

BEST PRACTICE FOR ALL

Expert decision-making in both medicine and nursing requires skills that cannot be quantified, and best practice often has outcomes which cannot be measured. However, the drive towards cost containment in healthcare and evidence that measurable targets have been met means that healthcare staff are likely to need to be able to justify the value of expertise. This includes how using expert staff who can weigh up all aspects of a situation, including the benefits of care protocols and clinical guidelines, rather than less expert staff who can follow guidelines and protocols with technical proficiency, is necessary and justifiable. The need to account for cost also applies to potentially justifying more expensive treatment and care than is recommended in national guidance when this is said to be in a patient's best interests. Thus, cost cannot be ignored by those seeking best practice. In the real world, best practice will be costly, and this cost will need to be justified.

Best practice includes providing care which best meets the needs of individual patients. It is therefore tempting to state that what the best interests of the individual patient are must be the concern of any healthcare professional at any given time, and to an extent this is true. However, in some respects it is an oversimplification of healthcare provision. No person stands in isolation, and the decisions made and actions taken in relation to one patient have inevitable effects on others. Healthcare is not an inexhaustible commodity, and thus healthcare professionals must take into account issues which are broader than one single patient. This is not to say that they should not do their utmost to determine the wishes and preferences of individual patients and to meet these as far as is possible. However, to practise in the real world means to practise within the reality that there are not enough resources to give everyone immediate access to their first choice of care. It is also likely that it will not be possible to provide every patient on every ward with immediate attention whenever they would like it. It is also sadly true that not everyone will act responsibly or consider others in their requests. Not everyone will make reasonable demands on the health service.

Although the well-being of every patient should be the prime concern of each practitioner in each individual encounter, the reality of healthcare is that there are many patients who need to be treated, and achieving best practice does not mean practising in an ivory tower, divorced from the realities of the competing demands of healthcare. Best practice includes being aware of the needs of individuals and groups, and, as well as weighing up the pros and cons of one aspect of care for one patient, it includes weighing up the care needs of groups of patients and the priorities within them. This requires greater expertise than managing a single patient encounter.

The reality is that healthcare professionals who state that they will only consider the best interests of each individual or what each individual patient wants in isolation are not working in the real world. They may provide what one patient considers being a high standard of care; however, they are unlikely to provide best care in the broader sense.

One approach to attempting to provide more equitable healthcare for all in a cost-constrained system has been the creation of clinical guidelines at a national level and the promise of national care protocols, to standardise what will be available. This has the potential to enhance the equality of care provision and to provide baseline standards of what should be provided. It may assist those seeking to produce best practice to work towards the complexity of providing best practice across the board, not just to individuals. However, in the same way that care protocols and clinical guidelines cannot replace expert practice in individual care situations, they cannot replace best practice across populations. They may be able to give guidance as to what are priorities and what patients can expect and what will be funded. They may even be necessary so that care is not provided on the basis of 'who shouts loudest gets'. However, they cannot perform the task of juggling the demands and needs of a range of patients so that the inevitable rationing which must occur in everyday practice is conducted to the highest level. They may give best recommendations for specific resources, and guidance on provision, but cannot guarantee best practice in resource allocation. For example, they may indicate when a patient with MS should usually be considered for treatment with interferon beta. However, they cannot assist a neurologist to determine how much time should be spent discussing diagnosis with a patient who has just been diagnosed with MS, compared to the time spent discussing the implications of disease with a young man who is losing the ability to walk as a result of disease progression, and carrying out assessment of another patient in whom neurological disease is suspected but not yet proven, within a finite amount of available time. Similarly, a care protocol may outline the procedures for preoperative care for a woman undergoing elective hysterectomy, but a protocol cannot determine how a nurse caring for six women in various pre- and postoperative stages on a gynaecology ward should divide her time between them.

To achieve best practice, clinical guidelines and care protocols must therefore be used as a guide on what is available and how certain approaches to care are best carried out. However, individual clinical expertise is still essential for individual patient care and the care of groups of patients and service management.

HOW HEALTHCARE PROFESSIONALS CAN INFLUENCE DECISION-MAKING

Healthcare professionals should aim to represent their patients' interests in decision-making. They have the rights of every citizen to representation via the ballot box, and their views on the politics surrounding healthcare will pre-sumably affect their voting behaviour.

In addition, as individual professions and joint professions, healthcare workers need to be aware of and involved in political debate. It is not enough to complain of politics and government influences on care in a manner which suggests that professional staff must be helpless bystanders. Healthcare pro-fessionals, not politicians, are the ones who are in day-to-day contact with patients, and frontline staff, not distant policymakers, are those who see patient care first-hand and know the challenges of this and how policy influences care. For practitioners to provide care based on the current best evidence, in the same way that evidence itself should be evaluated, healthcare policy and gov-ernment directives which influence care should be evaluated to ensure that they are indeed likely to promote the best care and to promote an effective use of resources.

Traditionally, medical staff have held the balance of power in healthcare. However, this appears to be altering. This may seem beneficial to staff groups who have traditionally held less power, and to patients. Nevertheless, health-care staff as a whole should be cautious that this change is used to give more equal power across professions and patients, not greater power to government and less representation of healthcare workers' or patients' views. While power shifts and changing roles in healthcare may be beneficial for patients, it is important that patients' quality of care remains central and that loss of power by one group of staff does not simply mean that distant politicians, not health-care professionals or patients, make the decisions.

There is an argument that nurses do not wish to engage in the politics of healthcare (Maslin-Prothero *et al.*, 2002). Nurses are the largest group of healthcare professionals, and arguably those who spend the most time with patients. They therefore have a professional responsibility to be involved in decision-making at local and national levels, and in representing the best inter-est of patients. Involvement in politics, at ward, local and national levels, is incumbent on professionals if best healthcare is to be available nationally. Of course not all nurses, midwives or medical staff can communicate directly with the Prime Minister, although it might be amusing if they did. However, all staff who are able to train as healthcare professionals should have the ability to at least consider the political implications of their practice. This can range from refusing to blindly accept instructions or a medical consultant's unexplained preferences and decisions, to questioning decision-making by Trust managers, to writing to local MPs and government departments about issues regarding care.

However, as challenging policy is not always likely to be welcome, health-care staff need to support each other at every level. This includes staff feeling that their colleagues, managers and governing bodies, as appropriate, will support them should their stance in seeking the best for their patients be dis-puted (Woodrow, 1997). This is not to say that every nurse and physician should be given carte blanche to be impossible to work with. Rather it means that, where policy or practice is challenged because an individual genuinely believes this to be in the patient's best interests, the philosophy behind this should be supported.

SUMMARY

In summary, then, clinical guidelines and care protocols give guidance. If this is good-quality guidance, following it has the potential to enhance care provision, provided this is done in a manner which is commensurate with the individual needs and preferences of patients, and that protocols or guidelines are not seen as the entirety of care provision. Best practice includes knowing when to follow guidelines or protocols, but also when not to.

Each individual patient is part of the larger picture of all patients for whom the finite healthcare resources of the NHS must be used. This is a part of real life, and healthcare staff who attempt to function without this consideration are unlikely to achieve best practice, although they may succeed in giving high-quality care to some individuals while possibly neglecting others. Difficult decisions must be made locally and nationally about how resources will be allocated, and this impacts upon the choices that are available to patients, and the time that care staff have to spend with them. Healthcare staff who aim to achieve best practice should not avoid such issues but should rather develop the skills needed to discuss realities of healthcare with patients so as to enable them to achieve the true autonomy which is informed choice, including information on the limits of a nationally funded service.

Best practice includes healthcare staff being aware of the political elements of their work and how their work is affected by political action. This includes national politics, local politics and interprofessional politics. Far from this detracting from patient care, any failure to be aware of political influences will adversely affect this care. It also requires a culture in which the questioning of the decisions of local and national policymakers by frontline staff is encouraged, rather than frowned upon. This is not something that will necessarily be welcomed by all parties, and particularly not by those whose power or authority is questioned. However, if healthcare professionals and patients, rather than government, are to be central to decision-making over healthcare, it is necessary. If healthcare professionals choose not to be involved in decision-making, be that at the frontline practice level of questioning local decisions or at the national level, they are not really entitled to complain about decisions made by others on their behalf.

Overall, then, clinical guidelines and care protocols are guidance, based on the best evidence, which state what is usually best. But for best practice, this information must be interpreted in individual circumstances. Guidance is only useful when it is used appropriately.

References

AGREE (2001) *AGREE Instrument*, The AGREE Collaboration, London.

Aiello, L.P., Brucker, A.J., Chang, S. *et al.* (2004) Evolving guidelines for intravitreous injections. *Retina*, 24 (5): S3–S19.

Antrobus, S. and Kitson, A. (1999) Nursing leadership: influencing and shaping health policy and nursing practice. *Journal of Advanced Nursing*, 29 (3): 746–53.

Arnsen, T.M. and Norheim, O.F. (2003) Quantifying quality of life for economic analysis: time out for time trade off. *Medical Humanities*, 29 (2): 81–6.

Bates, D.W., Kuperman, G.J., Wang, S. *et al.* (2003) Ten commandments for effective clinical decision support: making the practice of evidence based medicine a reality. *Journal of the American Informatics Association*, 10 (6): 523–30.

Beck, C.T. (2002) Postpartum depression: a metasynthesis. *Qualitative Health Research*, 12 (4): 453–72.

Bell, J. (2003) Resuscitating clinical research in the United Kingdom. *British Medical Journal*, 327 (7422): 1041–3.

Benner, P. (1984) *From Novice to Expert: Excellence and Power in Clinical Nursing Practice*, Addison Wesley Publishing, New York.

Benner, P. and Tanner, C. (1987) How expert nurses use intuition. *American Journal of Nursing*, 81 (1): 23–31.

Benner, P., Tanner, C. and Chesla, C. (1992) From beginner to expert: gaining a differentiated clinical world in critical care nursing. *Advances in Nursing Science*, 14 (3): 13–28.

Berenholtz, S. and Pronovost, P.J. (2003) Barriers to translating evidence into practice. *Current Opinion in Critical Care*, 9 (4): 321–5.

Bergus, G., Vogelgesang, S., Tansey, J. *et al.* (2004) Appraising and applying evidence about a diagnostic test during a performance based assessment, www.pubmedcentral. gov/articlerender.fcgi?tool=pubmed&pubmedid=15482600 (6 October 2005).

Bhandari, M., Montori, V., Devereaux, P.J. *et al.* (2003) Challenges to the practice of evidence-based medicine during residents' surgical training: a qualitative study using grounded theory. *Academic Medicine*, 78 (11): 1183–90.

Birch, S. and Gnafi, A (2003) NICE methodological guidelines and decision-making in the National Health Service in England and Wales. *Pharmacoeconomics*, 21 (3): 149–57.

Blank, R. and Burau, V. (2004) *Comparative Health Policy*, Palgrave, Basingstoke.

Boosfeld, B. and O'Toole, M. (2000) Technology dependent children: from hospital to home. *Paediatric Nursing*, 12 (6): 20–2.

Bridges, J., Hanson, R., Little, M. *et al.* (2001) Ethical relationships in paediatric emergency medicine: moving beyond the dyad. *Emergency Medicine*, 13 (3): 344–50.

Brinchmann, B.S., Forde, R. and Norvedt, P. (2002) What matters to parents? A qualitative study of parents' experiences with life-and-death decisions concerning their premature infants. *Nursing Ethics*, 9 (4): 388–404.

Brook, A. D., Ahrens, T. S. and Scaiff, R. (1999) Effect of a nurse implemented sedation protocol on duration of mechanical ventilation. *Critical Care Medicine*, 27 (12): 2609–15.

Brooks, N. and Barrett, A. (2003) Identifying nurse and health visitor priorities in a PCT using the Delphi technique. *British Journal of Community Nursing*, 8 (8): 376–80.

Bryson, B. (1997) *A Walk in the Woods*, Doubleday, London.

Buonocore, D. (2004) Leadership in Action: Creating Change in Practice. *AACN Clinical Issues: Advanced Practice in Acute and Critical Care*, 15 (2): 170–81.

Buss, L., Wlkinson, D. and Mitchell, R. (2004) Implementing a shared care: a dementia protocol, www.marc.soton.ac.uk/PDF%20FILES/LucySharedCarePublicationfinaldraft.pdf (7 October 2005).

Campbell, H., Hotchkiss, R., Bradshaw, N. and Porteous, M. (1998) Integrated care pathways. *British Medical Journal*, 316 (7125): 133–7.

Canter, R. (2001) Patients and medical power. *British Medical Journal*, 323 (7310): 41.

Caplan, A.L. (1992) *If I Were a Rich Man, Could I Buy a Pancreas?* Indiana University Press, Bloomington.

Caplan, I.R. (2001) Evidence-based medicine: concerns of a clinical neurologist. *Journal of Neurology, Neurosurgery and Psychiatry*, 71 (5): 569–74.

Cash, K. (1995) Benner and expertise in nursing: a critique. *International Journal of Nursing Studies*, 32 (6): 527–34.

CRD (2001) Undertaking Systematic Reviews of Research on Effectiveness. *CRD Report Number 4* (2nd edn).

Christiaens, T., De Backer, D., Burgers, J. and Baerheim, A. (2004) Guidelines, evidence and cultural factors. *Scandinavian Journal of Primary Healthcare*, 22 (3): 141–6.

Christiansen, M. and Hewitt-Taylor, J. (in press). Defining the expert ICU nurse. *Intensive and Critical Care Nursing*.

Clothier, C. (1994) *The Allitt Inquiry*, TSO, London.

Cochrane Collaboration (2005) *The Cochrane Manual* (issue 3). The Cochrane Collaboration, Oxford. www.cochrane.org/admin/manual.htm (4 August 2005).

Cole, A. and Shanley, E. (1998) Complementary therapies as a means of developing the scope of professional nursing practice. *Journal of Advanced Nursing*, 27 (6): 1171–6.

Considine, J. and Hood, K. (2000) Emergency department management of hip fractures: development of an evidence-based clinical guideline by literature review and consensus. *Emergency Medicine*, 12 (3): 329–36.

Coombes, R. (2005) NHS errors led to more than 800 deaths. *British Medical Journal*, 331 (7511): 254.

Coulter, A. (2002) After Bristol: putting patients at the centre. *British Medical Journal*, 324 (7338): 648–51.

Darbyshire, P. (1994) Skilled expert practice: is it 'all in the mind'? A response to English's critique of Benner's novice to expert model. *Journal of Advanced Nursing*, 19 (4): 755–61.

Davies, A.C.L. (2000) Don't trust me, I'm a doctor: medical regulation and the 1999 NHS reforms. *Oxford Journal of Legal Studies*, 20 (3): 437–56.

Davies, B.L. (2002) Sources and models for moving research evidence into clinical practice. *Journal of Obstetric Gynecological and Neonatal Nursing*, 31 (5): 558–62.

de Haes, H. and Koedoot, N. (2003) Patient-centred decision-making in palliative cancer treatment: a world of paradoxes. *Patient Education and Counseling*, 50 (1): 43–9.

DoH (1997) *A Bridge to the Future – Nursing Standards, Education and Workforce Planning in Paediatric Intensive Care*, DoH, London.

DoH (1998) *A First Class Service*, DoH, London.

DoH (2000) *The NHS Plan: a Plan for Investment, a Plan for Reform*, DoH, London.

DoH (2001) *The Expert Patient: a New Approach to Chronic Disease Management for the 21st Century*, DoH, London.

DoH (2002) *Delivering the NHS Plan*, DoH, London.

DoH (2003) *The NHS Knowledge and Skills Framework and Development Review Guidance: Working Draft*, DoH, London.

Department of Health and Social Security (1977) *The Extending Role of the Clinical Nurse – Legal Implications*, HMSO, London.

De Poy, E. and Gitlin, l. (1994) *Introduction to Research: Multiple Strategies for Health and Human Services*, Mosby, St. Louis.

Deshpande, N., Publicover, M., Gee, H. and Khan, K.S. (2003) Incorporating the views of obstetric clinicians in implementing evidence-supported labour and delivery suite ward rounds: a case study. *Health Information Library Journal*, 20 (2): 86–94.

Di Censo, A. Cullum, N. and Ciliska, D. (1998) Implementing evidence-based nursing: some misconceptions. *Evidence Based Nursing*, 1 (1): 38–9.

Diaz, J. (2004) Clinical reasoning in neurology. *Neurologia*, 36 (6, Supplement 1), 47–54.

Drake, R.E., Latimer, E.A., Leff, H.S. *et al.* (2004) What is evidence? *Child and Adolescent Psychiatric Clinics of North America*, 13 (4): 717–28.

Draper, H., Sorell, T. (2002) Patients' responsibilities in medical ethics. *Bioethics*, 16 (4): 335–52.

Dreyfus, H.L. and Dreyfus, S. (1980). A five-stage model of the mental activities involved in direct skill acquisition. University of California, Dissertation.

Dries, D.J., McGonigal, M.D., Malian, M.S., *et al.* (2004) Protocol driven ventilator weaning reduces use of mechanical ventilation, rate of early reintubation and ventilator associated pneumonia. *Journal of Trauma*, 56 (5): 943–51.

Dunn, N. (2002) Commentary: patient centred care: timely but is it practical? *British Medical Journal*, 324: 648–51.

Dyer, C. (2004) Hospital breached boy's human rights by treating him against his mother's wishes. *British Medical Journal*, 328 (7441): 661.

Dyer, C. (2005) Professor Roy Meadow struck off. *British Medical Journal*, 333 (7510): 177.

Edwards, A., Elwyn, G. and Mulley, A. (2002) Explaining risks: turning medical data into meaningful pictures. *British Medical Journal*, 324 (7341): 827–30.

Elstein, A.S. and Schwartz, A. (2002) Clinical problem solving and diagnostic decision-making: selective review of the cognitive literature. *British Medical Journal*, 324 (7339): 729–32.

Farrington, A. (1993) Intuition and expert clinical practice in nursing. *British Journal of Nursing*, 2 (4): 228–33.

Feasey, S. and Fox, C. (2001) Benchmarking evidence-based care. *Paediatric Nursing*, 13 (5): 22–5.

Feied, C.F., Handler, J.A., Smith, M.S. *et al.* (2004) Clinical information systems: instant ubiquitous clinical data error reduction and improved clinical outcomes. *Academy of Emergency Medicine*, 11 (11): 1162–9.

Fletcher, L. and Buka, P. (1999) *A Legal Framework for Caring*, Palgrave, Basingstoke.

Flottorp, S. and Oxman, A.D. (2003) Identifying barriers and tailoring interventions to improve the management of urinary tract infections and sore throat: a pragmatic study using qualitative methods. *Biomed Centre Health Service Research*, 3 (1): 3.

Freire, P. (1970) *Pedagogy of the Oppressed*, Penguin, London.

Frost, S., Crawford, P., Mera, S. and Chappell, B. (2003) Implementing good practice in epilepsy care. *Seizure*, 12 (2): 77–84.

Gallant, M.H., Beaulieu, M.C. and Carnevale, F.A. (2002) Partnership: an analysis of the concept within the nurse–client relationship. *Journal of Advanced Nursing*, 40 (2): 149–57.

Gartlehner, G., West, S.L., Lohr, K.N. *et al.* (2004) Assessing the need to update prevention guidelines: a comparison of two methods. *International Journal of Quality in Healthcare*, 16 (5): 399–406.

GMC (2000) Priorities and choices, www.gmc-uk.org/standards/priorities_and_choices. htm (25 May 2003).

General Medical Council (2005) The duties of a doctor registered with the General Medical Council, www.gmc-uk.org/standards/default.htm (4 August 2005).

Glendinning, C. and Kirk, S. (2000) 'High-tech care: high-skilled parents'. *Paediatric Nursing*, 12 (6), 25–7.

Gollop, R. (2003) Modernisation: fear of flying. *Health Service Journal*, 113 (5839): 28–9.

Goodman, N.W. (2000) Rational rationing. *British Medical Journal*, 321 (7272): 1356.

Gough, J. (2001) Public relations. *Nursing Standard*, 15 (26): 63.

Grace, P.J. (2001) Professional advocacy: widening the scope of accountability. *Nursing Philosophy*, 2 (2): 151–62.

Greenhalgh, T. (1999) Narrative-based medicine in an evidence-based world. *British Medical Journal*, 318 (7179): 323–5.

Griebsch, I., Coast, J. and Brown, J. (2005) Quality-adjusted life-years lack quality in pediatric care: a critical review of published cost-utility studies in child health. *Pediatrics*, 115 (5): 600–14.

Griffiths, F., Green, E. and Tsouroufli, M. (2005) The nature of medical evidence and its inherent uncertainty for the clinical consultation: a qualitative study. *British Medical Journal*, 330 (7490): 511.

Haddow, G. and Watts, R. (2003) Caring for a febrile child: the quality of Internet information. *Collegian*, 10 (2): 7–12.

Hall, S. (2001) Medical scandals leave trust in doctors unshaken. *Guardian*, 7 May 2001.

Harbour, R. and Miller, J. (2001) A new system for grading recommendations in evidence-based guidelines. *British Medical Journal*, 323 (7308): 334.

Heitkemper, M.M. and Bond, E.F. (2004) Clinical nurse specialists: state of the profession and challenges ahead. *Clinical Nurse Specialist*, 18 (3): 135–40.

Henderson, V. (1966) *The Nature of Nursing*, Collier–Macmillan, London.

Hewitt, J. (2002) A critical review of the arguments debating the roles of the nurse advocate. *Journal of Advanced Nursing*, 37 (5): 439–45.

Hewitt-Taylor, J. (2002) Case study: an approach to qualitative inquiry. *Nursing Standard*, 16 (2): 33–37.

Hewitt-Taylor, J. (2003) Evidence for practice. *Intensive and Critical Care Nursing*, 19 (2): 85–91.

Higuchi, K.A. and Donald, J.G. (2002) Thinking processes used by nurses in clinical decision-making. *Journal of Nurse Education*, 41 (4): 145–53.

Hu, W., Kemp, A. and Kerridge, I. (2004) Making clinical decisions when the stakes are high and the evidence unclear. *British Medical Journal*, 329 (7470): 852–4.

Hughes, M.S. (2002) Clinical Practice Guidelines, www.openclinical.org/guidelines.html (7 October 2005).

Jain, A. (2003) NICE recommends faster, easier access to care for MS patients. *British Medical Journal*, 327 (7426): 1247.

James, D.C., Simpson, K.R. and Knox, G.E. (2003) How do expert labor nurses view their role? *Journal of Obstetric Gynecological and Neonatal Nursing*, 32 (6): 814–23.

Joffe, S., Manocchia, M., Weeks, J.C. and Cleary, P.D. (2003) What do patients value in their hospital care? An empirical perspective on autonomy-centered bioethics. *Journal of Medical Ethics*, 29 (2): 103–8.

Johnson, M.E. and Hauser, P.M. (2001) The practices of expert psychiatric nurses: accompanying the patient to a calmer personal space. *Issues in Mental Health Nursing*, 22 (7): 651–68.

Jones, S. and Davies, J.S. (1999) The extended role of the nurse: the United Kingdom perspective. *International Journal of Nursing Practice*, 5 (4): 184–8.

Kaplan, C. (2002) Children and the law: the place of health professionals. Child and Adolescent. *Mental Health*, 7 (4): 181–8.

Kazanjian, A. (2001) How policy informs the evidence. *British Medical Journal*, 322 (7297): 1304.

Keaney, M. and Lorimer, A.R. (1999) Auditing the implementation of SIGN clinical guidelines. *International Journal of Healthcare Quality Assurance*, 12 (6–7): 314–7.

Kennedy, I. (2001) Learning from Bristol: the report of the public inquiry into children's heart surgery at the Bristol Royal Infirmary 1984–1995. Norwich, Bristol Inquiry Unit Cm. 5207, TSO, London.

Kennedy, I. (2003) Patients are experts in their own field. *British Medical Journal*, 326 (7402): 1276–77.

Kerrins, M.L. (2001) The advanced practice nurse role in paediatric home care. *Home Health Care Management and Practice*, 13 (5): 403–5.

Khan, F.A. and Hoda, M.Q. (2005) Drug-related critical incidents. *Anaesthesia*, 60 (1): 48–52.

King, L. and Clark, J.M. (2002) Intuition and the development of expertise in surgical ward and intensive care nurses. *Journal of Advanced Nursing*, 37 (4): 322–9.

King's Fund (2002) *The Future of the NHS: a Framework for Debate*, King's Fund, London.

Kneebone, R. and Darzi, A. (2005) New professional roles in surgery. *British Medical Journal*, 330 (7495): 803–4.

Kosko, B. (1994) *Fuzzy Thinking*, HarperCollins, London.

Lancaster, T., Sheppard, S. and Silgay, C. (1997) Systematic reviews and meta-analysis, in *Assessment and Evaluation of Health and Medical Care* (eds J. Dowie, T. Lancaster, S. Sheppard and C. Silgay), Open University Press, Buckingham, pp. 171–83.

Lawrie, S.M., Scott, A.I. and Sharpe, M.C. (2000) Evidence-based psychiatry – do psychiatrists want it and can they do it? *Health Bulletin*, 58 (1): 25–33.

Leninger, M.M. (1991) *Culture Care Diversity and Universality: a Theory of Nursing*, National League of Nursing Press, New York.

Lewis, S.J. and Orland, B.I. (2004) The importance and impact of evidence-based medicine. *Journal of Managed Care Pharmacy*, 10 (5, Suppl. A): S3–5.

Liberati, A., D'Amico, R., Pifferi, S. *et al.* (2002) *Antibiotics for Preventing Respiratory Tract Infections in Adults Receiving Intensive Care*, (Cochrane Review, Issue 3), The Cochrane Library, Oxford.

Lincoln, Y.S. and Guba, E.G. (1986) But is it rigorous? Trustworthiness and authenticity in naturalistic evaluation. *New Directions Program Evaluation*, 30 (1): 73–84.

Littlejohns, P., Leng, G., Culyer, T. and Drummond, M. (2004) NICE clinical guidelines: maybe health economists should participate in guideline development. *British Medical Journal*, 329 (7465): 571.

Livesey, A. (2005) A multiagency protocol for responding to sudden unexpected death in infancy: descriptive study. *British Medical Journal*, 330 (7485): 227–8.

Long, L.E. (2003) Imbedding quality improvement into all aspects of nursing practice. *International Journal of Nursing Practice*, 9 (5): 280–4.

Loss, J. and Nagel, E. (2005) Does evidence-based surgery harm autonomy in clinical decision-making? *Zentralbl Chir*, 130 (1): 1–6.

Lowden, J. (2002) Children's rights: a decade of dispute. *Journal of Advanced Nursing*, 37 (1): 100–7.

Maiden, V. and Hewitt-Taylor, J. (2005) Linking theory and practice in children's nursing: lessons from abroad. *Paediatric Nursing*, 17 (5): 24–8.

Martin, C. (2002) The theory of critical thinking of nursing. *Nursing Education Perspectives*, 23 (5): 243–7.

Martin, G. (1998) Ritual action and its effect on the nurse as advocate. *Journal of Advanced Nursing*, 27 (1): 189–94.

Maslin-Prothero, S. Ed, C. and Masterson, A. (2002) Power, politics, and nursing in the United Kingdom. *Policy, Politics, and Nursing Practice*, 3 (2): 108–17.

Max, A., Gattuso, J. and Hinds, P. *et al.* (2003) Developing nursing care guidelines for children with Hodgkin's disease. *European Journal of Oncology Nursing*, 7 (4): 253–8.

MacDonald, M. and Bodzak, W. (1999) The performance of a self-managing day surgery nurse team. *Journal of Advanced Nursing*, 29 (4): 859–68.

McCance, T.V., McKenna, H.P. and Boore, J.R.P. (1999) Caring: theoretical perspectives of relevance to nursing. *Journal of Advanced Nursing*, 30 (6): 1388–95.

McKendry, M., McGloin, H. and Saberi, D. et al. (2004) Randomised controlled trial for assessing the impact of a nurse-delivered, flow-monitored protocol for the optimisation of circulatory status after cardiac surgery. *British Medical Journal*, 329 (7460): 258.

McKinlay, E., McLeod, D., Dowell, A. and Marshall, C. (2004) Clinical practice guidelines' development and use in New Zealand: an evolving process. *New Zealand Medical Journal*, 117 (1199): U999.

Meerabeau, L. (1992) Tacit nursing knowledge: an untapped resource or a methodological headache? *Journal of Advanced Nursing*, 17 (1): 108–12.
Michie, S. and Johnston, M. (2004) Changing clinical behaviour by making guidelines specific. *British Medical Journal*, 328 (7435): 343–5.
Miners, A.H., Garau, M., Fidan, D. and Fischer, A.J. (2005) Comparing estimates of cost effectiveness submitted to the National Institute of Clinical Excellence (NICE) by different organisations: a retrospective study. *British Medical Journal*, 330 (7482): 65.
Moore, T. (2005) After the fall. *Financial Times Magazine*, 9–10 July 2005, p. 8.
Moore, W. (1970) *The Professions*, Russell Sage Foundation, New York.
Morris, A.H. (2001) Rational use of computerised protocols in the intensive care unit. *Critical Care*, 5 (5): 249–54.
Mohanty, K.C. (2005) Influence of guidelines in determining medical negligence. *British Medical Journal*, 330 (7499): 1086–7.
Mulhall, A. (1998) Nursing research and the evidence. *Evidence Based Nursing*, 1 (1): 4–6.
Mulhall, A., Kelly, D. and Pearce, S. (2001) Naturalistic approaches to healthcare evaluation: the case of a teenage cancer unit. *Journal of Clinical Excellence*, 3 (4): 167–73.
Muminovic, M. (2002) Calculating risks. *British Medical Journal*, 325 (7363): 552a.
National Health and Medical Research Council (2000) *How to Put Evidence into Practice*, National Health and Medical Research Council, Canberra.
National Electronic Library for Health (2005) About integrated care pathways, www.libraries.nelh.nhs.uk/pathways/aboutICPs.asp (4 August 2005).
NHS Modernisation Agency and NICE (2004a) What is protocol-based care? www.modern.nhs.uk/protocolbasedcare/whatis_leaflet.pdf (7 October 2005).
NHS Modernisation Agency and NICE (2004b) A step-by-step guide to developing protocols, www.modern.nhs.uk/protocolbasedcare/step2step.pdf (7 October 2005).
NICE (2000) Arrhythmias – implantable cardioverter defibrillators (ICDs) (No. 11), NICE, London.
NICE (2001) Guidance on the use of cyclo-oxygenase (Cox) II selective inhibitors, celecoxib, rofecoxib, meloxican and etodolac for osteoarthritis and rheumatoid arthritis, www.nice.org.uk/page.aspx?o=18034 (7 October 2005).
NICE (2002b) Type 2 diabetes – blood glucose, G, NICE, London.
NICE (2002c) Type 2 diabetes – management of blood pressure and blood lipids, H, NICE, London.
NICE (2002d) Type 2 diabetes – renal disease, F, NICE, London.
NICE (2002e) Type 2 diabetes – retinopathy, E, NICE, London.
NICE (2002f) Smoking cessation – bupropion and nicotine replacement therapy (No. 39), NICE, London.
NICE (2002g) Beta interferon and glatiramer acetate for the treatment of multiple sclerosis. Technology Appraisal Guidance no. 32, NICE, London.
NICE (2003a) Chronic heart failure, CG5, NICE, London.
NICE (2003b) Pancreatic islet cell transplantation, IPG013, NICE, London.
NICE (2003c) Microwave endometrial ablation, IPG 007, NICE, London.
NICE (2003d) Antenatal care, CG6, NICE, London.
NICE (2003e) Multiple sclerosis, CG8, NICE, London.
NICE (2003f) Preoperative tests, CG3, NICE, London.
NICE (2003g) Head injury, CG4, NICE, London.
NICE (2004a) Sepsis (severe) – drotrecogin (No. 84), NICE, London.

NICE (2004b) Dyspepsia, CG17, NICE, London.
NICE (2004c) Self-harm, CG16, NICE, London.
NICE (2004d) Depression, CG23, NICE, London.
NICE (2004e) Epilepsy, CG20, NICE, London.
NICE (2004f) Type 2 diabetes: footcare, CG10, NICE, London.
NICE (2004g) Type 1 diabetes, CG15, NICE, London.
NICE (2004h) Caesarean section, CG13, NICE, London.
NICE (2004i) Framework document, www.nice.org.uk/page.aspx?o=219813 (6 August 2005).
NICE (2004j) The guideline development process: an overview for stakeholders, the public and the NHS, www.nice.org.uk/pdf/GDP_An_Overview_for_Stakeholders_the_Public_and_the_NHS.pdf (7 October 2005).
NICE (2005a) Holding statement – European review of safety of Cox II inhibitors, www.nice.org.uk/pdf/CoxII_holdingstatement.pdf (7 October 2005).
NICE (2005b) Clinical guidelines, www.nice.org.uk/page.aspx?o=cg (6 August 2005).
NICE (2005c) Lung cancer, CG 24, NICE, London.
Nelson, A.M. (2002) A metasynthesis: mothering other-than-normal children. *Qualitative Health Research*, 12 (4): 515–30.
Norheim, O.F. (1999) Healthcare rationing: are additional criteria needed for assessing evidence-based clinical practice guidelines? *British Medical Journal*, 319 (7222): 1426–9.
NMC (2002) *The Code of Professional Practice*, NMC, London.
O'Connor, A.M., Llewellyn-Thomas, H.A. and Flood, A.B. (2004) Modifying unwarranted variations in healthcare: shared decision making using patient decision aids http://content.healthaffairs.org/cgi/content/abstract/hlthaff.var.63(1) (6 October 2005).
Oxford English Dictionary (2001) *Oxford English Dictionary*, Oxford University Press, Oxford.
Pagliari, C. and Grimshaw, J. (2002) Impact of group structure and process on multidisciplinary evidence-based guideline development: an observational study. *Journal of Evaluation of Clinical Practice*, 8 (2): 145–53.
Paul, W.P. and Heaslip, P. (1995) Critical thinking and intuitive nursing practice. *Journal of Advanced Nursing*, 22 (1): 40–7.
Plouffe, J. and Seniuk, C. (2004) Walking the walk: living evidence-based practice. *Dynamics*, 15 (1): 14–17.
Popay, J., Rogers, A. and Williams, G. (1998) Rationale and standards and the review of qualitative literature in health services research. *Qualitative Health Care Research*, 8 (3): 341–51.
Poses, R.M. (2003) A cautionary tale: the dysfunction of American healthcare. *European Journal of Internal Medicine*, 14 (2): 123–30.
Poulter, N.R. (2004) NICE and BHS guidelines on hypertension differ importantly. *British Medical Journal*, 329 (7477): 1289.
Pritchard, M., Flenady, V. and Woodgate, P. (2002) *Preoxygenation for Tracheal Suctioning in Intubated, Ventilated Newborn Infants* (Cochrane Review, issue 3), The Cochrane Library, Oxford.
Protheroe, J., Fahey, T., Montgomery, A.A. and Peters, T.J. (2000) The impact of patients' preferences on the treatment of atrial fibrillation: observational study of patient-based decision analysis. *British Medical Journal*, 320 (7246): 1380–4.

Radwin, L. (1995) Knowing the patient: a process model for individualised interventions. *Nursing Research*, 44 (6): 364–70.

Rawlins, M.D., Lipman, T., Hart, J.T. *et al.* (2001) The failings of NICE. *British Medical Journal*, 322 (7284): 489.

Rawlins, R.P., William, S.R. and Beck, C.C. (1993) *Mental Health – Psychiatric Nursing: a Holistic Life-cycle Approach*, 3rd edn, Mosby, London.

Redfern, S. and Christian, S. (2003) Achieving change in healthcare practice. *Journal of Evaluation in Clinical Practice*, 9 (2): 225–38.

Ricart, M., Lorente, C., Diaz, E. and Kollef, M.H. (2003) Nursing adherence with evidence-based guidelines for preventing ventilator-associated pneumonia. *Journal of Critical Care Medicine*, 31 (11): 2693–6.

Riley, R. and Peters, G. (2000) The current scope and future direction of perioperative nursing practice in Victoria, Australia. *Journal of Advanced Nursing*, 32 (3): 544–53.

Rolfe, G. (1996) Closing the theory–practice gap: a model of nursing praxis. *Journal of Clinical Nursing*, 6 (2): 173–7.

Rolfe, G. (1997) Science, abduction and the fuzzy nurse: an exploration of expertise. *Journal of Advanced Nursing*, 25 (6): 1070–5.

Rosenthal, J., Rymer, J., Jones, R. *et al.* (2005) Chaperones for intimate examinations: cross-sectional survey of attitudes and practices of general practitioners. *British Medical Journal*, 330 (7485): 234–5.

RCN (1998) *Clinical Practice Guidelines: the Management of Patients with Venous Leg Ulcers*, RCN, London.

RCN (2001) *Pressure Ulcer Risk Assessment and Prevention*, RCN, London.

RCN (2003) *Defining Nursing*, RCN, London.

Ryan, J., Piercy, J. and James, P. (2004) Assessment of NICE guidance on two surgical procedures. *Lancet*, 363 (9420): 1525–6.

Rycroft-Malone, J. (2001) Formal consensus: the development of a national clinical guideline. *Quality Healthcare*, 10 (4): 238–44.

Sackett, D.L., Rosenberg, W.M.C., Gray, J.A.M. *et al.* (1996) Evidence-based medicine: what it is and what it isn't. *British Medical Journal*, 312 (7023): 71–2.

Salter, B. (2001) Who rules? The new politics of medical regulation. *Social Science and Medicine*, 52 (6): 871–83.

Schulkin, J. (2000) Decision sciences and evidence-based medicine – two intellectual movements to support clinical decision-making. *Academic Medicine*, 75 (8): 816–18.

SIGN (2002a) *Prevention and Management of Hip Fracture in Older People.* SIGN 56, SIGN, Edinburgh.

SIGN (2002b) *Cardiac Rehabilitation.* SIGN 57, SIGN, Edinburgh.

SIGN (2003a) *Management of Obesity in Children and Young People.* SIGN 69, SIGN, Edinburgh.

SIGN (2003b) *Epithelial Ovarian Cancer.* SIGN 75, SIGN, Edinburgh.

SIGN (2004a) *A Guideline Developer's Handbook.* SIGN 59, SIGN, Edinburgh.

SIGN (2004b) *Management of Osteoporosis.* SIGN 71, SIGN, Edinburgh.

SIGN (2005) SIGN and NICE: Working together to improve patient care, www.sign.ac.uk/about/niceandsign.html (30 September 2005).

Scott, I., Heyworth, R. and Fairweather, P. (2000) The use of evidence-based medicine in the practice of consultant physicians: results of a questionnaire survey. *Australian and New Zealand Journal of Medicine*, 30 (3): 319–26.

Scott, P.A. (2003) Allocation of resources: an issue for nurses, in *Ethics in Nursing Education, Research and Management* (ed W. Tadd), Palgrave, Basingstoke, pp. 145–62.

Semin-Goossens, A., van der Helm, J.M. and Bossuyt, P.M. (2003) A failed model-based attempt to implement an evidence-based nursing guideline for fall prevention. *Journal of Nursing Care Quarterly*, 18 (3): 217–25.

Shannon, C. (2003) Money must be made available for NICE guidance, minister says. *British Medical Journal*, 327 (7428): 1368–a.

Shaw, J. and Barker, M. (2004) 'Expert Patient': Dream or Nightmare? *British Medical Journal*, 328 (7442): 723–4.

Sheldon, T.A., Cullum, N., Dawson, D. *et al.* (2004) What's the evidence that NICE guidelines have been implemented? *British Medical Journal*, 329 (7473): 1003–4.

Silagy, C.A., Stead, F. and Lancaster, T. (2001) Use of systematic reviews in clinical practice guidelines: a case study of smoking cessation. *British Medical Journal*, 323: 833–6.

Smeeth, L. (2000) Commentary: patients, preferences, and evidence. *British Medical Journal*, 320 (7246): 1384.

Smith, J. (2005) *Shipman Report*, HMSO, London.

Smith, R. (2003) Need good results? Fiddle them. *British Medical Journal*, 326 (7398): 1048.

Stewart, P.M. (2003) Improving clinical research. *British Medical Journal*, 327 (7422): 999–1000.

Stoykova, B., Drummond, M., Barbieri, M. and Kleijnen, J. (2003) The lag between effectiveness and cost-effectiveness evidence of new drugs. Implications for decision-making in healthcare. *European Journal of Health Economics* 4 (4): 313–18.

Sullivan, M. (2003) The new subjective medicine: taking the patient's point of view on healthcare and health. *Social Science and Medicine*, 56 (7): 1595–604.

Thomas, D.E., Kukuruzovic, R., Martino, B. *et al.* (2003) Knowledge and use of evidence-based nutrition: a survey of paediatric dietitians. *Journal of Human Nutrition and Dietetics*, 16 (5): 315–22.

Thomas, L. (1999) Clinical practice guidelines. *Evidence Based Nursing*, 29 (2): 38–9.

Thompson, P. (2000) Implementing evidence-based healthcare: the nurse teacher's role in supporting the dissemination and implementation of SIGN clinical guidelines. *Nurse Education Today*, 20 (3): 207–17.

Thorne, S., Paterson, B., Acorn, S. *et al.* (2002) Chronic illness experience: insights from a metastudy. *Qualitative Health Research*, 12 (4) 437–52.

Tracy, C.S., Dantas, G.C. and Upshur, R.E. (2003) Evidence-based medicine in primary care: qualitative study of family physicians. *Biomed Central Family Practitioner*, 4 (1): 6.

Tweedale, M.G. (2002) Grasping the nettle – what to do when patients withdraw their consent for treatment: (a clinical perspective on the case of Ms B). *Journal of Medical Ethics*, 28 (4): 236–7.

UKCC (1992) *The Scope of Professional Practice*, UKCC, London (now The Nursing and Midwifery Council).

Wailoo, A., Roberts, J., Brazier, J. and McCabe, C. (2004) Efficiency, equity, and NICE clinical guidelines. *British Medical Journal*, 328 (7439): 536–7.

Wall, R.J., Dittus, R.S. and Ely, E.W. (2001) Protocol-driven care in the intensive care unit: a tool for quality. *Critical Care*, 5 (6): 283–5.

Warne, T. and McAndrew, S. (2004) Mirror mirror on the wall, who is the most improved of all? *Journal of Nursing Management*, 12 (2): 131–6.

Wathen, B. and Dean, T. (2004) An evaluation of the impact of NICE guidance on GP prescribing. *British Journal of General Practice*, 54 (499): 103–7.

Watson, J. (1985) *Nursing: Human Science and Human Care – a Theory of Nursing*, The National League of Nursing Press, New York.

Weissman, S.H. (2000) The need to teach a wider, more complex view of evidence. *Academic Medicine*, 75 (10): 957–8.

Wilcox, R.A. and Whitham, E.M. (2003) Reduction of medical error at the point of care using electronic clinical information delivery. *International Medical Journal*, 33 (11): 537–40.

Wilkin, K. (2002) Exploring expert practice through reflection. *Nursing in Critical Care*, 7 (2): 88–93.

Wilmot, S. (2003) *Ethics, Power and Policy: the Future of Nursing in the NHS*, Palgrave, Basingstoke.

Winyard, G. (2003) Doctors, managers and politicians. *Clinical Medicine*, 3 (5): 465–9.

Witkin, S.L. and Harrison, W.D. (2001) Whose evidence and for what purpose? *Social Work*, 46 (4): 293–5.

Wolfson, R.K., Kahana, M.D., Nachman, B. and Lantos, J. (2005) Extracorporeal membrane oxygenation after stem cell transplant: clinical decision-making in the absence of evidence. Pediatric *Critical Care Medicine*, 6 (2): 200–3.

Woodrow, P. (1997) Nurse advocacy: is it in the patient's best interests? *British Journal of Nursing*, 6. (4): 225–9.

Woolery, L. (1990) Expert nurse and expert systems. *Computers in Nursing*, 8 (1): 23–7.

Wyatt, J.C. Paterson-Brown, S., Johanson, R. *et al.* (1998) Randomised trial of educational visits to enhance use of systematic reviews in 25 obstetric units. *British Medical Journal*, 317 (7165): 1041–6.

Index